Guidelines for
NUTRITION CARE OF RENAL PATIENTS
Third Edition

Kerri L. Wiggins, MS, RD

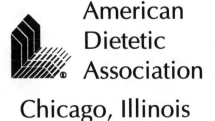

American
Dietetic
Association

Chicago, Illinois

Library of Congress Cataloging-in-Publication Data

Wiggins, Kerri Lynn.

Guidelines for nutrition care of renal patients / Kerri L. Wiggins.—3rd ed.

p. ; cm.

"A project of the Renal Dietitians Dietetic Practice Group of the American Dietetic Association."

Rev. ed. of: Suggested guidelines for nutrition care of renal patients / editors, Katy G. Wilkens, Katherine Brouns Schiro, 2nd ed. c1992.

Includes bibliographical references and index.

ISBN 0-88091-189-1

1. Chronic renal failure—Nutritional aspects. 2. Chronic renal failure—Diet therapy.

I. American Dietetic Association. Renal Practice Group. II. Suggested guidelines for nutrition care of renal patients.

[DNLM: 1. Nutrition Assessment. 2. Kidney Failure, Chronic—diet therapy. WJ 342 W655g 2001]

RC918.R4W496 2001

616.6'140654—dc21   2001033287

The views expressed in this publication are those of the authors and do not necessarily reflect policies and/or official positions of the American Dietetic Association. Mention of product names in this publication does not constitute endorsement by the authors or the American Dietetic Association. The American Dietetic Association disclaims responsibility for the application of the information contained herein.

10 9 8 7 6 5 4 3 2

Contents

Preface

The field of renal nutrition continues to change rapidly. When advances in the science of renal disease and its complications occur, health care practices must be altered to keep pace with them. To stay current with these changes, and to support the important work of dietetics professionals, *Guidelines for Nutrition Care of Renal Patients,* third edition, has been completely revised and updated.

The guidelines have been a valuable resource for renal dietitians since their introduction in 1986 by the Renal Dietitians Dietetic Practice Group (RPG) of the American Dietetic Association. Reviewed and field-tested by a nationwide committee of renal dietitians, the guidelines established criteria for optimal nutritional care of renal patients and promoted consistency among the practices of nutrition practitioners. This third edition of the guidelines has been developed to follow the American Dietetic Association's Medical Nutrition Therapy (MNT) Protocol format to further assist dietitians in consistently providing optimal care to renal patients. These guidelines define the appropriate level, content, and frequency of nutrition care based on the best available scientific information and expert opinion; they provide a framework to assist the dietitian in the assessment, intervention, and evaluation of outcomes for MNT. As MNT protocols, the guidelines can also be used to facilitate the measurement of the quality and effectiveness of nutrition care.

With this revision, a number of changes have been made to the original guidelines. *Guidelines for the Care of Adult Dialysis In-Center Patients* and *Guidelines for the Care of Adult Home Dialysis Patients* have been combined in *Guideline 2, Nutrition Care of Adult Dialysis Patients.* The *Guidelines for Nutrition Care of Hospitalized Adult Renal Transplant Patients* have been expanded to become *Guideline 6, Nutrition Care of Transplant Patients*, and now include pretransplant evaluation and nutrition care for both acute and chronic stages posttransplantation. With the increased incidence of successful pregnancies in renal patients within the past few years and the increase in practitioner experience in caring for these patients, it was possible to field-test the guidelines for pregnant renal patients published in this edition. The previous sections on *Nutrition Care of Pregnant Dialysis Patients*, *Nutrition Care of Pregnant Patients With Renal Insufficiency*, and *Nutrition Care of Pregnant Patients With Renal Transplant* are now integrated into the *Guideline 7, Nutrition Care of Adult Pregnant ESRD Patients.*

This revision contains two new sections: *Guideline 5, Nutrition Care of Adult Acute Renal Failure Patients* is provided to delineate the appropriate level of nutrition care for patients hospitalized with the diagnosis of acute renal failure. *Guideline 3, Enteral/Parenteral Nutrition Support of Adult Dialysis Patients* defines the appropriate level of nutrition care for dialysis patients, cared for in an outpatient dialysis center or at home, who receive tube-feeding or parenteral nutrition support.

Each of the guidelines presented here was researched, written, reviewed, and field-tested by registered dietitians from throughout the United States. All were written to complement the National Kidney Foundation's Dialysis Outcomes Quality Initiative (NKF-DOQI) clinical practice guidelines, a set of guidelines developed to improve patient outcomes by providing recommendations for the optimal medical care of renal patients. In addition, several members of the NKF-DOQI committees reviewed and provided input on the revised guidelines.

Acknowledgments

This publication is the result of countless hours of work by dedicated professionals—the editors and reviewers who contributed their time and expertise to make this publication what it is. We wish to thank the following persons who helped to review and field-test the guidelines:

Debbie Alexandrowcz, RD
Linda Aytona, MA, RD
Margaret Baker, RD, CNSD
Julie Barbosa, MS, RD, CNSD, CSR
Wendy Barrett, MS, RD
Matilda Barron, RD, CSR, CD
Diane Bell, ScD, RD
Thelma Blew, MS, RD
Rebecca Bradley, RD
Wendy Bratz, RD
Carol Burns, MS, RD
Jerrilyn Burrowes, MS, RD, CDN, CSR
Paige Cady, RD
Sarah Carter, RD, CDE
Ann Cave, RD
Janice Chapman, MS, RD, LD
Flora Chen, MS, RD, CSR
Carolyn Cochran, MS, RD, LD
Connie Crawford, MS, RD, CSR
Carol Cunningham, MS, RD
Alysun Deckert, MS, RD
Linda DeNering, MS, RD
Ann Cooper Erb, RD, CSR
Lori Fedje, RD, LD
Martha Ference, RD
Betty Fisher, MS, RD
Geralyn Gilotti, RD
Cathy Goeddeke-Merickel, MS, RD
Laura Griffiths, MS, RD, LD
Erleen Hamlin, RD
Marsha Herke, MPH, RD
Jennifer Hernon, RD
Geri Jennings, RD, CD

Marcia Kalista-Richards, MS, RD, CNSD
Beverly Kastan, MS, RD
Susan Knapp, MS, RD
Andrew Levy, MD
Susan Lewis, RD, CNSD
Jill Lindberg, MD, FACP
Ann Lipkin, MS, RD
Jenny Lipo, RD
Marty Loeffler, RD, CSR, LD
Marge Magness, RD, CSR
Elizabeth Mask, RD
Linda McCann, RD, LD
Maureen McCarthy, MPH, RD, CSR
Steve Montaya, MD
Fay Moore, RD, CSR
Joni Pagenkemper, MS, MA, RD
Mark Parker, MD
Chhaya Patel, MA, RD
Jessie Pavlinac, MS, RD, CSR, LD
Jan Peiffer, RD, LN
Terry Rydzon, RD, CSR
Laura Sabban, MS, RD
Sharon Schatz, MS, RD, CSR, CDE
Charla Schultz, RD, LD
Cathy Seifert, RD
Linda Snetselaar, PhD, RD
Robin Taber, RD, CNSD
Ann Twork, MS, RD
Cydney Wolf, RD
Marsha Wolfson, MD, FACP
Ester Wong, RD, LD
Laura Ann Yates, MS, RD, LD

Introduction

Overview   These guidelines have been developed to assist dietitians in providing efficient and effective nutrition care for patients with kidney disease and in evaluating outcomes of the medical nutrition therapy (MNT) provided. The guidelines are meant to serve as a general framework for handling patients with particular health problems. It may not always be appropriate to use these guidelines to manage patients. Individual circumstances vary and can require actions that differ from these guidelines. For example, different treatment may be appropriate for patients who are severely ill or who have comorbid, socioeconomic, or other complicating conditions. The independent skill and judgement of the health care provider must always dictate treatment decisions. These guidelines are provided with the express understanding that they do not establish or specify particular standards of care, whether legal, medical, or other.

The guidelines have been designed for specified care settings as designated at the beginning of each section, and treatment of patients in other care settings will require a deviation from the guidelines. Most of the guidelines have been written for care provided in the outpatient setting, including dialysis facilities and extended care facilities. In particular, the *Guidelines for Enteral/Parenteral Nutrition Support of Adult Dialysis Patients* are for patients treated at an outpatient dialysis center or with home dialysis, and are not meant to be used with hospitalized dialysis patients. For dialysis patients requiring inpatient tube feeding and/or parenteral nutrition, more appropriate guidelines can be found in the enteral and parenteral medical nutrition therapy guidelines published by the American Dietetic Association's Dietitians in Nutrition Support Practice Group. The guidelines that are not written for the outpatient setting are the *Guidelines for Nutrition Care of Adult Hospitalized Dialysis Patients, Guidelines for Nutrition Care of Acute Renal Failure Patients*, and the "Acute Phase" in the *Guidelines for Nutrition Care of Transplant Patients*.

Provision of care may need to progress from one guideline to another depending on the patient's medical status, the current treatment mode, and the patient's disease progression. For example, a patient may begin receiving care under the Pre-ESRD guidelines, but then, if the patient progresses to requiring dialysis treatment, the patient would need to be followed using the dialysis guidelines. If the same patient received a transplant, care would continue using the Transplant guidelines.

Comments from the review process indicated that some reviewers found parts of the guidelines repetitive and too detailed. However, although many skilled services that dietitians provide are assumed or appear minor, it is critical that all processes involved in nutritional assessment and intervention be delineated in order to document the extensive and comprehensive care that renal dietitians provide.

Organization of the Guidelines

The format of the guidelines has been changed to maintain consistency with Medical Nutrition Therapy Protocols that have been developed and to improve the provision of care and evaluation of patient outcomes. The guidelines follow the Sample Medical Nutrition Therapy Protocol format developed by the American Dietetic Association.

Each guideline is organized into a minimum of five sections, with some having additional sections. The first three sections delineate care provided by the dietitian and expected patient outcomes and may be useful for managed care organizations (MCOs), administrators, and other health care providers.

Section 1: Synopsis/Summary

This section summarizes the patient population to which the guideline pertains and includes diagnosis, age, and type of care setting. For chart audit purposes, situations in which the guidelines do not apply are noted as *Exceptions*. The number of encounters, the expected length of time for each contact, and the time frame between encounters is also listed. The expected length of time incorporates the time spent reviewing information prior to seeing the patient, assessing the patient, providing intervention, documenting the intervention, and the time needed for any other duties required to provide appropriate MNT for the patient. The *Intervals Between Encounters* defines the point in time at which each encounter should be completed following the previous encounter.

Section 2: Process Flowchart

The flowchart visually depicts the process of interventions, the types of data to be obtained, and the necessary time frames. The individual encounters, with the time at which the assessment and intervention should be completed, are listed on the left side of the flowchart. Data to be obtained during the assessment and intervention stages corresponding to each encounter are listed on the right.

Section 3: Expected Outcomes of Medical Nutrition Therapy

The tables in this section summarize the outcomes expected as a result of the MNT provided. The Outcome Assessment Factors are divided into two major categories: *Clinical Outcomes* and *Patient/Caregiver Behavioral Outcomes*. Clinical outcomes include anatomic and physiologic measures such as biochemical parameters, anthropometrics, and clinical signs and symptoms. Behavioral outcomes include measures of change in the patient's (or caregiver's) behavior, as related to food selection, food preparation, and activity, which will ultimately result in change in clinical and/or functional outcomes. It is important to stress that these outcomes are patient-oriented, not dietitian-oriented.

The *Expected Outcome of Therapy* indicates the type of change anticipated as a result of MNT provided, such as increasing, decreasing, or stabilization of laboratory values.

The *Ideal/Goal Value* column lists the values, as defined in the literature, that are considered appropriate for control or improvement of patient nutritional status.

Section 4: Session Descriptives

In this last section, *Minimum Baseline Data* tables include information that is needed by the dietitian prior to the initial encounter with the patient. This information may be obtained from a variety of sources, including the patient chart and other health professionals.

Each guideline contains several individual session descriptives. In general each guideline contains an *Initial Session* which covers the first visit with the patient and a *Follow-up Session* which, in some cases, is repeated at the indicated intervals. The guidelines for Pre-ESRD, Dialysis, and Enteral/Parenteral Nutrition Support also contain *Nutritional Updates* which are routine interventions to be carried out at the interval that is specified. The Hospitalized Dialysis and Acute Renal Failure guidelines contain a *Discharge Planning* section to be completed prior to the patient's discharge. Because of the multiple stages involved in transplantation, Guidelines for Nutrition Care of Transplant Patients is organized into three sections according to patient or transplant status. The *Pretransplant Evaluation* is provided for the initial nutritional evaluation prior to the patient receiving a transplant. As this is typically a one-time visit, no Follow-up Session is included. The posttransplant *Acute Phase* and *Chronic Phase* both contain Initial and Follow-up Sessions. The three sections can be used independently of each other.

The individual sessions contain two major divisions: an *Assessment* table and an *Intervention* table. The session length at the top of each table refers to the total time needed to complete both the assessment and the intervention and to document the intervention appropriately. The *Assessment* table contains, primarily, information obtained from the patient during the patient interview and information used to assess nutritional status that must be determined by the dietitian. Some elements included in this table, such as psychosocial and economic issues, may be assessed by other health-care team members and can be obtained from them. The *Intervention* table reflects the response of the dietitian to the assessment information, and includes calculation of the patient's nutritional needs, counseling of the patient according to the assessed educational needs, and communication with the other members of the health care team.

Section 5: Bibliography

Each guideline includes a bibliography of the references used in the development of the section.

Guideline Specifics

Pre-ESRD

- Evaluates the patient needing nutritional counseling but not yet requiring dialysis treatment.

Dialysis

- Encompasses patients receiving dialysis in a dialysis center or at home via either hemodialysis or peritoneal dialysis.
- In-center hemodialysis patients are routinely followed by the dialysis facility's dietitian with counseling and interventions provided on an on-going basis. Laboratory values and patient status are typically monitored on a monthly basis with interventions made in response to aberrant labs.

Enteral/Parenteral Nutrition Support in Dialysis

- Designed for patients receiving dialysis at an outpatient dialysis center or at home, and not meant to be used with hospitalized dialysis patients. For dialysis patients requiring inpatient tube-feeding and/or parenteral nutrition, refer to the nutrition support specialist or team within the hospital.
- Enteral nutrition in these guidelines refers to tube-feeding and the term "formula" refers to either enteral or parenteral formulas.

Hospitalized Dialysis

- A guide for care of the dialysis patient in the hospital setting.
- These guidelines are not meant to replace Joint Commission on Accreditation of Healthcare Organizations (JCAHO) guidelines.
- Specifics for nutrition support are not delineated in this guideline. For patients requiring nutrition support, refer to the nutrition support specialist or team within the hospital.
- The nutrition care presented in this guideline may not all be provided within the hospital setting. A patient may be discharged to an extended care or rehabilitation facility, and then the patient care and education would continue in that setting.

Acute Renal Failure

- To be utilized with patients diagnosed with acute renal failure in the hospital setting.
- These guidelines are not meant to replace Joint Commission on Accreditation of Healthcare Organizations (JCAHO) guidelines.
- Specifics for nutrition support are not delineated in this guideline. For patients requiring nutrition support, refer to the nutrition support specialist or team within the hospital.

- The nutrition care presented in this guideline may not all be provided within the hospital setting. A patient may be discharged to an extended care or rehabilitation facility, and then the patient care and education would continue in that setting.

Transplant

- Includes three stages of transplantation: Pretransplant, Acute Posttransplant, and Chronic Posttransplant. The three sections can be used independently of each other.

Pregnant ESRD

- Covers pregnancy in the pre-ESRD patient, the dialysis patient, and the transplant patient.

Source

Medical Nutrition Therapy Across the Continuum of Care. Chicago, Ill: The American Dietetic Association; 1996.

Guideline 1
Nutrition Care of Adult Pre-ESRD Patients

Synopsis/Summary

Diagnosis: Renal Insufficiency, including nephrotic syndrome (Adult 18+ years)

Setting: Ambulatory Care

Exceptions for Chart Audit: Patients who are younger than 18 years of age; patients who begin dialysis, receive a transplant, or die within 1 month; patients who do not keep appointments. For subjective data, patients who are unwilling or unable to communicate and have no caregivers who wish to do so.

Encounter	Length of Contact	Intervals Between Encounters
Initial	60–90 minutes	Within 1 month of referral
Follow-up	30–45 minutes	3–4 weeks, or as determined necessary
Nutritional Updates	45–60 minutes	Quarterly

Adult Pre-ESRD Flowchart

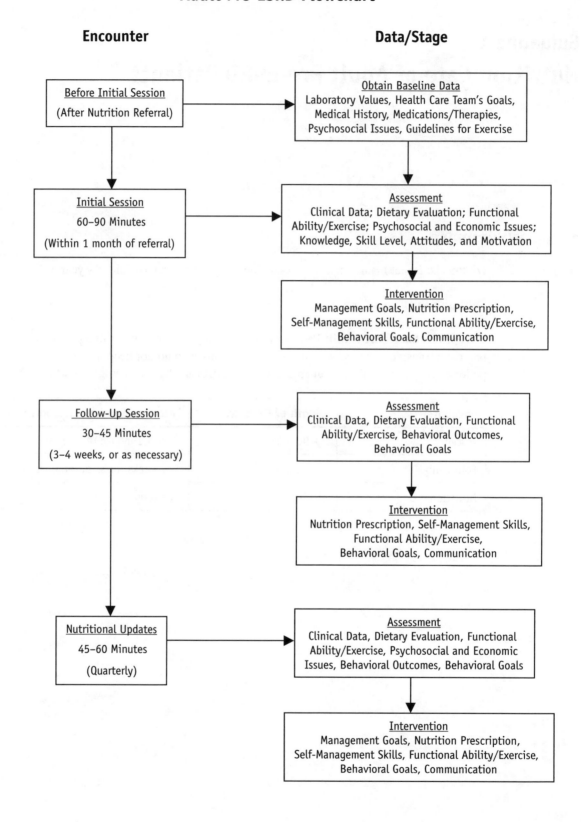

Encounter

Data/Stage

Before Initial Session
(After Nutrition Referral)

Obtain Baseline Data
Laboratory Values, Health Care Team's Goals,
Medical History, Medications/Therapies,
Psychosocial Issues, Guidelines for Exercise

Initial Session
60–90 Minutes
(Within 1 month of referral)

Assessment
Clinical Data; Dietary Evaluation; Functional
Ability/Exercise; Psychosocial and Economic Issues;
Knowledge, Skill Level, Attitudes, and Motivation

Intervention
Management Goals, Nutrition Prescription,
Self-Management Skills, Functional Ability/Exercise,
Behavioral Goals, Communication

Follow-Up Session
30–45 Minutes
(3–4 weeks, or as necessary)

Assessment
Clinical Data, Dietary Evaluation, Functional
Ability/Exercise, Behavioral Outcomes,
Behavioral Goals

Intervention
Nutrition Prescription, Self-Management Skills,
Functional Ability/Exercise,
Behavioral Goals, Communication

Nutritional Updates
45–60 Minutes
(Quarterly)

Assessment
Clinical Data, Dietary Evaluation, Functional
Ability/Exercise, Psychosocial and Economic
Issues, Behavioral Outcomes, Behavioral Goals

Intervention
Management Goals, Nutrition Prescription,
Self-Management Skills, Functional Ability/Exercise,
Behavioral Goals, Communication

Expected Outcomes of Medical Nutrition Therapy

Outcome Assessment Factors	Expected Outcome of Therapy	Ideal/Goal Value
Clinical Outcomes • Biochemical Parameters — BUN, creatinine — Albumin — Potassium — Phosphorus — Calcium — Serum glucose (premeal) — HbA1c (diabetes) — Cholesterol — Triglycerides (fasting) — Creatinine clearance/GFR	**Measure < 30 days prior to nutrition session** —BUN and creatinine levels stabilized —Albumin maintained within goal range (stabilized in nephrotic syndrome) —Potassium maintained within goal range —Phosphorus and calcium progressing toward goal ranges —Blood sugar levels maintained within goal range —Cholesterol and triglyceride levels progressing toward goal ranges —Decline in creatinine clearance/GFR minimized	 —BUN and creatinine levels stabilized —Albumin 3.5–5.0 g/dL (may be lower in nephrotic syndrome) —Potassium 3.5–5.5 mEq/l —Phosphorus 2.5–5.0 mg/dL —Calcium 8.5–10.5 mg/dL —Serum glucose 80–120 mg/dL —HbA1c < 7 % —Cholesterol 120–240 mg/dL —Triglycerides < 200 mg/dL —Creatinine clearance/GFR stabilized
• Hematological Parameters —Hematocrit/Hemoglobin —Ferritin —Transferrin saturation • Anthropometrics —Weight • Clinical Signs and Symptoms	—Adequate erythropoiesis maintained —Adequate iron stores maintained for erythropoiesis —Reasonable weight achieved/maintained —Adequate body mass maintained —Level of functional ability maintained —Good appetite maintained —Appropriate blood pressure control maintained	—Hematocrit 33–36% hemoglobin 11.0–12.0 g/dL —Ferritin 100–800 ng/ml —Transferrin saturation 20%–50% —Within reasonable body weight (BMI 20–25) —Adequate muscle/fat stores —Optimum functional ability —Minimum GI symptoms —Food intake > 80% recommended intake —Blood pressure within appropriate limits
Patient/Caregiver Behavioral Outcomes • Food selection/meal planning • Nutrient needs • Potential food/drug interactions • Exercise	—Exhibits positive changes in food selection and amounts —If diabetic, times meals and snacks appropriately —Identifies foods with a significant protein content —Verbalizes potential food/drug interactions —If no medical limitations, gradually increases or continues physical activity level	**MNT Goals** 1. Makes appropriate food choices and takes medications as prescribed 2. Maintains appropriate protein intake 3. Maintains lab values within acceptable limits 4. If diabetic, maintains stable glucose levels through appropriate dietary practices. 5. If no medical limitations, maintenance of an exercise program.

Minimum Baseline Data Needed for MNT

Factor	Data Needed
Laboratory Values with Dates (within 30 days of session)	1. BUN, creatinine 2. Albumin 3. Sodium, potassium, phosphorus, calcium 4. Serum glucose 5. Lipid profile 6. Serum bicarbonate 7. PTH, if available 8. Hematocrit/hemoglobin 9. Ferritin, transferrin saturation 10. Urinalysis results (e.g., volume, urea, protein, sodium) 11. Creatinine clearance or GFR 12. Others as appropriate (e.g., glycosylated hemoglobin)
Health Care Team Goals for Patient	1. Patient prognosis, expected onset of dialysis 2. Expected outcome of nutrition therapy
Medical History	1. Disease/condition causing renal insufficiency 2. History of renal disease and treatment 3. Concurrent medical conditions (e.g., diabetes, cancer, HIV, cardiovascular disease, GI problems, hypertension, hyperlipidemia) 4. Any other medical or physical conditions with potential nutritional implications (e.g., surgery, infection, CVA, chemotherapy, blindness, neuropathies)
Medications/Therapies	1. Diet order, tube feeding order, and/or parenteral nutrition order 2. Any other treatments or therapies that may affect nutritional intake or status 3. Antihypertensives, diuretics 4. Phosphate binders 5. Vitamin/mineral supplements 6. Any other medications with food/drug interactions or nutritional impact (e.g., diabetes medications, GI medications, steroids)
Psychosocial Issues	1. Learning disabilities 2. Vision, hearing abilities 3. Cultural or language barriers 4. Mental status
Guidelines for Exercise	1. Medical clearance for exercise 2. Exercise limitations, if any

Initial Nutrition Assessment

Session: *Initial*   Length: *60–90 minutes*   Time: *Within 1 month of referral*

Factor	Assessments
Clinical Data	1. Review Minimum Baseline Data table. 2. Obtain current height, weight, and BMI. 3. Obtain weight history, recent weight changes, and weight goals. 4. Determine IBW and/or UBW adjusted for amputation or obesity, and percentage IBW and/or percentage UBW (see Appendix B). 5. Assess muscle and fat stores, presence of edema. 6. Assess for physical signs of nutrient deficiencies/excesses or increased needs (e.g., decubiti, poor wound healing, thinning hair, pale conjunctiva, cheilosis). 7. Determine nitrogen balance using urea kinetics, if appropriate (see Appendix D). 8. Assess blood pressure control.
Dietary Evaluation	1. Determine previous dietary instruction and practices. 2. Determine usual food intake and pattern of intake. 3. Assess appetite, GI issues, tolerance of oral intake, and food allergies/intolerances. 4. Assess feeding issues (e.g., chewing, swallowing). 5. Determine use of vitamin/mineral, herbal, or other nutrition supplements. 6. Determine alcohol/drug/tobacco use and history. 7. Assess intake of calories, protein, sodium, and other nutrients as indicated (e.g., carbohydrates, fats, potassium, phosphorus, calcium, and fluids). 8. Assess diet order, tube feeding order, and/or parenteral nutrition order for appropriateness.
Functional Ability/Exercise	1. Determine level of functional ability and recent changes. 2. Assess ability to feed self and needs for assistance. 3. Determine activity level and exercise habits. 4. Determine physical or motivational limitations to exercise.
Psychosocial and Economic Issues	1. Assess living situation, cooking facilities, finances, educational background, employment, literacy, and other factors that may affect availability of food. 2. Assess ethnic or religious belief considerations. 3. Assess availability of support systems. 4. Determine whether other relevant psychosocial or economic issues exist.
Knowledge, Skill Level, Attitudes, and Motivation	1. Assess basic knowledge level of dietary guidelines for renal insufficiency. 2. Assess basic knowledge level of impact of renal insufficiency on nutrition. 3. Assess attitudes toward nutrition and health. 4. Determine patient's willingness and ability to learn and make appropriate changes.

Initial Nutrition Intervention

Session: *Initial*   Length: *60–90 minutes*   Time: *Within 1 month of referral*

Factor	Interventions
Management Goals	1. Identify management goals of health care team. 2. Identify patient goals and expectations.
Nutrition Prescription	1. Calories-individualized to maintain reasonable weight; use basal energy expenditure x activity factor (1.2–1.3) x stress factor; or use > 35 kcal/kg IBW or adjusted weight 2. Protein-based on creatinine clearance, GFR, urinary protein losses (0.6–1.0 g/kg IBW or adjusted weight), 50% from high biological value animal and/or plant sources 3. Fats-for lipid abnormalities: fats, cholesterol, and carbohydrates adjusted per severity of risk factors (see Appendixes G and H) 4. Sodium-individualized, or 1–3 g/day 5. Potassium-individualized per lab values 6. Phosphorus-individualized, or 8–12 mg/kg IBW or adjusted weight; may require phosphate binder therapy 7. Calcium-individualized per calcium, phosphorus, and PTH lab values; use of vitamin D; and supplementation level 8. Fluids-as desired to maintain appropriate hydration status 9. Vitamin/mineral supplementation-as appropriate
Self-Management Skills	1. Discuss simple definitions and examples of calories, protein, sodium, and other nutrients as appropriate (e.g., carbohydrates, fats, potassium, phosphorus, calcium, fluids). 2. Discuss basic dietary guidelines for renal insufficiency. 3. For diabetes, discuss basic dietary guidelines and timing of meals and snacks, if indicated. 4. Discuss laboratory tests and significance of results. 5. Discuss use and effect of phosphate binders, if prescribed. 6. Discuss food/drug interactions as indicated. 7. Discuss role and effect of diet and medications on renal function. 8. Discuss role of blood pressure control and blood glucose regulation in slowing the progression of renal failure. 9. Assess comprehension of education provided and projected compliance.
Functional Ability/Exercise	1. Provide necessary referrals for assistance with self-feeding and other activities of daily living (e.g., OT, PT, speech therapy). 2. Discuss exercise recommendations, if appropriate.
Behavioral Goals	1. Address eating and exercise behaviors. 2. Identify and summarize short-term behavioral goals that are specific and achievable. 3. Establish follow-up plan.
Communication	1. Document current nutritional status, plan of care, and goals of MNT. 2. Report recommendations/concerns to appropriate health care team member (e.g., MD, RN, pharmacist, social worker). 3. Provide information regarding nutrition prescription and dietary guidelines to referral source, extended-care facility, home health care agencies, if appropriate.

Follow-up Nutrition Assessment

Session: *Follow-up*   Length: *30–45 minutes*   Time: *3–4 weeks, or as necessary*

Factor	Assessments
Clinical Data	1. Review changes in medical status and recent/planned therapies (e.g., medications, surgery). 2. Review any new or updated laboratory data. 3. Assess changes in weight. 4. Assess muscle and fat stores, presence of edema. 5. Assess for physical signs of nutrient deficiencies/excesses or increased needs (e.g., decubiti, poor wound healing, thinning hair, pale conjunctiva, cheilosis) 6. Assess blood pressure control. 7. Assess effectiveness of previous nutrition intervention.
Dietary Evaluation	1. Determine current GI or feeding issues or concerns. 2. Assess changes in patient's food intake and/or appetite. 3. Assess dietary intake and/or nutritional support intake for adequacy and appropriateness.
Functional Ability/Exercise	1. Assess changes in functional ability. 2. Assess changes in activity level or exercise habits.
Behavioral Outcomes	1. Assess understanding of simple definitions and examples of calories, protein, sodium, and other nutrients as appropriate (e.g., carbohydrates, fats, potassium, phosphorus, calcium, fluids). 2. Assess understanding of basic dietary guidelines for renal insufficiency. 3. For diabetes, assess understanding of basic dietary guidelines and timing of meals and snacks. 4. Assess understanding of laboratory tests and significance of results. 5. Assess understanding of use and effect of phosphate binders. 6. Assess understanding of food/drug interactions. 7. Assess understanding of role and effect of diet and medications on renal function. 8. Assess understanding of role of blood pressure control and blood glucose regulation in slowing the progression of renal failure. 9. Determine further improvements that can be made in the quality of the diet.
Behavioral Goals	1. Assess achievement of prior behavioral goals. 2. Determine willingness and ability to make further changes.

Follow-up Nutrition Intervention

Session: *Follow-up*   Length: *30–45 minutes*   Time: *3–4 weeks, or as necessary*

Factor	Interventions
Nutrition Prescription	1. Provide feedback on lab results, blood pressure control, changes in weight. 2. Provide feedback on food/meal plan, food choices and portions. 3. Recommend changes in nutrient intake or habits that may improve outcomes. 4. Adjust MNT, as is appropriate.
Self-Management Skills	1. Review and reinforce self-management skills from first session. 2. Provide and review educational materials as appropriate. 3. If medications change, discuss potential food/drug interaction. 4. Assess comprehension of education provided and projected adherence.
Functional Ability/Exercise	1. Refer to OT, PT, speech therapy as is appropriate. 2. Discuss changes in exercise recommendations, if appropriate.
Behavioral Goals	1. Reset short-term behavioral goals that are specific and achievable. 2. Review and reinforce long-term goals. 3. Establish follow-up plan.
Communication	1. Document current nutritional status, plan of care, and goals of MNT. 2. Report recommendations/concerns to appropriate health care team member (e.g., MD, RN, pharmacist, social worker). 3. Provide information regarding nutrition prescription and dietary guidelines to referral source, extended-care facility, home health care agencies, if appropriate.

Quarterly Nutrition Assessment

Session: *Nutritional Update*   Length: *45–60 minutes*   Time: *Quarterly*

Factor	Assessments
Clinical Data	1. Review changes in medical status and recent/planned therapies (e.g., medications, surgery). 2. Review recent laboratory data. 3. Assess changes in weight. 4. Determine BMI, IBW, and/or UBW adjusted for amputation or obesity, and percentage IBW and/or percentage UBW (see Appendix B). 5. Assess muscle and fat stores, presence of edema. 6. Assess for physical signs of nutrient deficiencies or excesses (e.g., decubiti, poor wound healing, thinning hair, pale conjunctiva, cheilosis). 7. Determine nitrogen balance using urea kinetics (see Appendix D). 8. Assess blood pressure control. 9. Assess effectiveness of previous nutrition intervention.
Dietary Evaluation	1. Determine current GI or feeding issues or concerns, tolerance of oral intake. 2. Assess changes in patient's food intake and/or appetite. 3. Determine use of vitamin/mineral, herbal, or other nutrition supplements. 4. Assess intake of calories, protein, sodium and other nutrients as indicated (e.g., carbohydrates, potassium, phosphorus, calcium, and fluids). 5. Assess diet order, tube feeding order, and/or parenteral nutrition order for appropriateness.
Functional Ability/Exercise	1. Determine level of functional ability and recent changes. 2. Assess ability to feed self and needs for assistance. 3. Assess changes in activity level or exercise habits. 4. Determine physical or motivational limitations to exercise.
Psychosocial and Economic Issues	1. Assess changes in living situation, cooking facilities, finances, education, employment, literacy, and other factors which may affect availability of food. 2. Assess availability of support systems. 3. Determine if other relevant psychosocial or economic issues exist.
Behavioral Outcomes	1. Assess understanding of prior nutrition education and food/meal plan. 2. Assess appropriateness of food intake and pattern of intake. 3. Assess understanding of relevant food/drug interactions. 4. Determine further improvements that can be made in the quality of the diet.
Behavioral Goals	1. Assess achievement of prior behavioral goals. 2. Determine willingness and ability to make further changes.

Quarterly Nutrition Intervention

Session: *Nutritional Update*   Length: *45–60 minutes*   Time: *Quarterly*

Factor	Interventions
Management Goals	1. Reassess and adjust management goals of patient and health care team.
Nutrition Prescription/ Feedback	1. Provide feedback on lab results, blood pressure control, changes in weight. 2. Provide feedback on food/meal plan, food choices and portions. 3. Recommend changes in nutrient intake or habits that may improve outcomes. 4. Adjust MNT, as is appropriate.
Self-Management Skills	1. Review and reinforce self-management skills. 2. Provide and review educational materials as is appropriate. 3. If medication change, discuss potential food/drug interaction. 4. Assess comprehension of education provided and projected compliance.
Functional Ability/Exercise	1. Provide necessary referrals for assistance with self-feeding and other activities of daily living (e.g., OT, PT, speech therapy). 2. Discuss changes in exercise recommendations, if appropriate.
Behavioral Goals	1. Reset short-term behavioral goals that are specific and achievable. 2. Review and reinforce long-term goals. 3. Establish follow-up plan.
Communication	1. Document current nutritional status, plan of care, and goals of MNT. 2. Report recommendations/concerns to appropriate health care team member (e.g., MD, RN, pharmacist, social worker). 3. Provide information regarding nutrition prescription and dietary guidelines to referral source, extended-care facility, home health care agencies, if appropriate.

Bibliography

American Diabetes Association Position Statement: Diabetic Nephropathy. *DiabetesCare.* 1997; 20(Suppl 1):S24–S27.

American Diabetes Association Position Statement: Hospital Admission Guidelines for Diabetes Mellitus. *DiabetesCare.* 1997; 20(Suppl 1):S52.

American Diabetes Association Position Statement: Implications of the Diabetes Control and Complications Trial. *DiabetesCare.* 1997; 20(Suppl 1):S62–S64.

American Diabetes Association Position Statement: Nutrition Recommendations and Principles for People with Diabetes Mellitus. *Diabetes Care.* 1997; 20(Suppl 1):S14–S17.

American Diabetes Association Position Statement: Screening for Diabetes. *DiabetesCare.* 1997; 20(Suppl 1):S22–S23.

American Diabetes Association Position Statement: Standards of Medical Care for Patients with Diabetes Mellitus. *DiabetesCare.* 1997; 20(Suppl 1):S5–S13.

American Diabetes Association. *Maximizing the Role of Nutrition in Diabetes Management.* Alexandria, Va: American Diabetes Association, Inc; 1994.

Attman PO, Alaupovic P. The role of lipid metabolism in dietary treatment of chronic renal failure. *ContribNephrol.* 1990; 81:35–41.

Attman PO, Alaupovic P. Dietary treatment of uraemia and the relation to lipoprotein metabolism. *EuroJClinNutr.* 1992;46:687–696.

Attman PO, Alaupovic P. Lipid abnormalities in chronic renal insufficiency. *KidneyInt.* 1991 39(Suppl 31):S16–S23.

Avram MM, Sreedhara R, Avram DK, Muchnick RA, Fein P. Enrollment parathyroid hormone level is a new marker of survival in hemodialysis and peritoneal dialysis therapy for uremia. *AmJKidneyDiseases.*1996; 28(6): 924–930.

Bargman JM. The rationale and ultimate limitations of urea kinetic modelling in the estimation of nutritional status. *PeritonealDialysisInt.* 1996; 16:347–351.

Barsotti G, Cupisti A, Morelli E, Meola M, Giovannetti S. Dietary treatment of Type I diabetic nephropathy with renal insufficiency. In Guarnieri G, Panzetta G, Toigo G (eds). Metabolic and nutritional abnormalities in kidney disease. *ContribNephrology.* 1992; 98:149–156.

Beto JA. Which diet for which renal failure: Making sense of the options. *JAmDietAssoc.* 1995; 95(8):898–903.

Beto JA. Highlights of the consensus conference on prevention of progression in chronic renal disease: implications for dietetic practice. *JRenalNutr.* 1994; 4(3):122–126.

Bianchi ML, Colantonio G, Campanini F, Rossi R, Valenti G, Ortolani S, Buccianti G. Calcitriol and Calcium carbonate therapy in early chronic renal failure. *Nephrol Dial Transplant.* 9:1595–1599,1994.

Bourke E, Delaney V. Assessment of hypocalcemia and hypercalcemia. *Clin LabMed.* 1993; 13(1):157–181.

Breyer JA. Therapeutic interventions for nephropathy in Type I diabetes mellitus. *SeminNephrol.* 1997; 17(2):114–123.

Bucciante G, Senesi G, Piva M, et al. Resting metabolic rate by indirect calorimetry in uremic patients. In Albertazzi A, Cappelli P, Del Rosso G, Di Paolo B, Evangelista M, Palmieri PF (eds). Nutritional and pharmacological strategies in chronic renal failure. *ContribNephrology.* 1990; 81:214–219.

Cappuccio FP, MacGregor GA. Dietary salt restriction: Benefits for cardiovascular disease and beyond. *CurrOpinNephrolHypertension.* 1997; 6:477–482.

Carvalho AB, Lobao RRS, Cuppari L, Draibe SA, Ajzen H. Does hypophosphataemia induce hypoparathyroidism in pre-dialysis patients? *NephrolDialTransplant.* 1998; 13(Suppl 3):12–14.

Castaneda C, Grossi L, Dwyer J. Potential benefits of resistance exercise training on nutritional status in renal failure. *JRenalNutr*. 1998; 8(1):2–10.

Castaneda C. The relationship between rehabilitation and nutrition status in renal disease patients. *Contemp Dial & Neph* Aug:18–21,1997.

Chicago Dietetic Association, South Suburban Dietetic Association, Dietitians of Canada. *Manual of Clinical Dietetics* (6th ed). Chicago: American Dietetic Association;1996.

Cianciaruso B, Bellizzi V, Minutolo R, et al. Salt intake and renal outcome in patients with progressive renal disease. *MinerElectrolyteMetab*. 1998; 24:296–301.

D'Amico G, Gentile MG. Pharmacological and dietary treatment of lipid abnormalities in nephrotic patients. *KidneyInt*. 1991; 39(Suppl 31):S65–S69.

D'Amico G, Gentile MG. Effect of dietary manipulation on the lipid abnormalities and urinary protein Loss in nephrotic patients. *MinerElectrolyteMetab*. 1992; 18:203–206.

Daugirdas JT, Ing TS. *Handbook of Dialysis* (2nd ed). Boston:Little, Brown and Company; 1994.

Delmez JA, Slatopolsky E. Hyperphosphatemia: Its consequences and treatment in patients with chronic renal disease. *AmJKidneyDis*. 1992; 19(4):303–317

Dureke TB, Barany P, Cazzola M, et al. Management of iron deficiency in renal anemia: guidelines for the optimal therapeutic approach in erythropoietin-treated patients. *ClinNephrol*. 1997; 48(1):1–8.

Farkas-Hirsch R (ed). *Intensive Diabetes Management*. Alexandria, Va: American Diabetes Association; 1995.

Fishbane S, Maesaka JK. Iron management in end-stage renal disease. *AmJKidneyDis*. 1997; 29(3):319–333.

Foley RN, Parfrey PS. Anemia in predialysis chronic renal failure: What are we treating? *JamSocNephrol*. 1998; 9:S82–S84.

Gillis BP, Caggiula AW, Chiavacci AT, et al. Nutrition intervention program of the modification of diet in renal disease study: A self-management approach. *JAmDietAssoc*. 1995; 95(11):1288–1294.

Glassock RJ, Cohen AH, Adler SG. Primary glomerular diseases. In Brenner BM (ed). *Brenner and Rector's The Kidney* (5th ed). Philadelphia, Pa: WB Saunders Co; 1996.

Grant A, DeHoog S. *Nutritional Assessment and Support* (5th ed). Seattle, Wa: Anne Grant/Susan DeHoog; 1991.

Gretz N, Strauch M. Protein Restriction and progression of chronic renal failure. *EuroJClinNutr*. 1992; 46:765–772.

Henrich WL. Approach to volume control, cardiac preservation, and blood pressure control in the pre-end-stage renal disease patient. *JAmSocNephrol*. 1998; 9:S63–S65.

Hirschberg RR, Kopple JD. Energy requirements in patients with renal failure. *ContribNephrol*. 1990; 81:124–135.

Hirshberg RR, Kopple JD. Energy requirements in patients with renal failure. In Albertazzi A, Cappelli P, Del Rosso G, Di Paolo B, Evangelista M, Palmieri PF (eds). Nutritional and pharmacological strategies in chronic renal failure. *ContribNephrology*. 1990; 81:124–135.

Irvin B. The renal application of the 1994 Diabetes Guidelines. *JRenalNutr*. 1997; 7(3):158–161.

Irvin B. Nutrition in the prevention and progression of diabetic nephropathy. *RenalNutrForum*. 1997; 16(1):1–4,22.

Irvin B. The progression and treatment of diabetic nephropathy. *TopClinNutr*. 1996; 12(1):31–40.

Kasiske BL. Hyperlipidemia in patients with chronic renal disease. *AmJKidneyDis*. 1998; 32(5, Suppl 3):S142–S156.

Kaysen GA. Nutritional management of nephrotic syndrome. *JRenalNutr*. 1992; 2(2):50–58.

Keane WF, Mulcahy WS, Kasiske BL, Kim Y, O'Donnell MP. Hyperlipidemia and progressive renal disease. *KidneyInt*. 1991; 39(Suppl 31):S41–S48.

Klahr S, Levey AS, Beck GJ, et al. The effects of dietary protein restriction and blood-pressure control on the progression of chronic renal disease. *NewEngJMed*. 1994; 350(13):877–884.

Klahr S, The MDRD Study Group. Primary and secondary results of the modification of diet in renal disease study. *MinerElectrolyteMetab*. 1996; 22:138–142.

Kopple JD, Massry SG (eds). *Nutritional Management of Renal Disease*. Baltimore: Williams & Wilkins; 1997.

Lebovitz HE (ed). *Therapy for Diabetes Mellitus and Related Disorders* (2nd ed). Alexandria, Va,:American Diabetes Association, Inc.; 1994.

Levey AS, Hakim RM. The pros and cons of protein restriction for dialysis patients are debated. *ContempDialNeph*. 1997; Aug:16–17.

Levey AS. Controlling the epidemic of cardiovascular disease in chronic renal disease: Where do we start? *AmJKidneyDis*. 1998; 32(5,Suppl 3):S5–S13.

Levine DZ (ed). *Care of the Renal Patient* (2nd ed). Philadelphia: W.B. Saunders Company; 1991.

Mackenzie HS, Brenner BM. Current strategies for retarding progression of renal disease. *AmJKidneyDis*. 1998; 31(1):161–170.

Mailloux LU, Levey AS. Hypertension in patients with chronic renal disease. *AmJKidneyDis*. 1998;32(5,Suppl 3):S120–S141.

Malluche HH, Monier-Faugere MC. Uremic bone disease: Current knowledge, controversial issues, and new horizons. *MinerElectrolyteMetab*. 1991;17:281–296.

Manske CL. Hyperglycemia and intensive glycemic control in diabetic patients with chronic renal disease. *AmJKidneyDis*. 1998; 32(5,Suppl 3):S157–S171.

Maroni BJ. Nutrition in the predialysis patient. *DialTransplant*. 1994; 23(2):76–83,94.

Maroni BJ. Protein restriction in the pre-end-stage renal disease (ESRD) patient: Who, when , how, and the effect on subequent ESRD outcome. *JamSocNephro*. 1998; 9:S100–S106.

Maschio G, Oldrizzi L, Rugiu C, De Biase V, Loschiavo C. Effect of dietary manipulation on the lipid abnormalities in patients with chronic renal failure. *KidneyInt*. 1991; 39(Suppl 31):S70–S72.

McCann L (ed). *Pocket Guide to Nutritional Assessment of the Adult Renal Patient* (2nd ed). New York: National Kidney Foundation; 1998.

Messa P, Vallone C, Mioni G, Geatti O, Turrin D, Passoni N,et al. Direct in vivo assessment of parathyroid hormone-calcium relationship curve in renal patients. *KidneyInt*. 1994; 46:1713–1720.

Mitch WE, Maroni BJ. Nutritional considerations and the indications for dialysis. *AmJKidneyDis*. 1998; 31(1):185–189.

Mitch WE, Maroni BJ. Nutritional considerations in the treatment of patients with chronic uremia. *MinerElectrolyteMetab*. 1998; 24:285–289.

Mitch WE, Walser M. Nutritional therapy for the uremic patient. In Brenner BM (ed). *Brenner and Rector's The Kidney* (5th ed). Philadelphia: WB Saunders Co;1996.

Mitch WE. Influence of metabolic acidosis on nutrition. *AmJKidneyDis*. 1997; 9(5):xivi-xiviii.

Mitch WE. Low-protein diets in the treatment of chronic renal failure. *JamCollNutr*. 1995; 14(4):311–316.

Mitch WE. Mechanisms causing muscle wasting in uremia. *JRenalNutr*.1996; 6(2):75–78.

Modification of diet in renal disease study group. Effects of dietary protein restriction on the progression of moderate renal disease in the modification of diet in renal disease study. *JAmSoNephrol*. 1996; 7(12):2616–2626.

Molitch ME. The relationship between glucose control and the development of diabetic nephropathy in Type I diabetes. *SeminNephrol*. 1997; 17(2):101–113.

Morbidity and Mortality of Dialysis. NIH Consensus Statement. 1993; Nov 1–3 11(2):1–33.

Nissenson AR. Achieving target hematocrit in dialysis patients: New concepts in iron management. *AmJKidneyDis*. 1997; 30(6):907–911.

NKF-DOQI Clinical Practice Guidelines for the Treatment of Anemia of Chronic Renal Failure. New York: National Kidney Foundation; 1997.

Nordal KP, Dahl E, Halse J, Attramadal A, Flatmark A. Long-term low-dose calcitriol treatment in predialysis chronic renal failure: can it prevent hyperparathyroid bone disease? *NephrolDial-Transplant*. 1995; 10:203–206.

Oldrizzi L, Rugiu C, Maschio G. Nutrition and the kidney: How to manage patients with renal failure. *NutrClinPract*. 1994.; 9:3–10.

Olmer M, Pain D, Dussol B, Berland Y. Protein diet and nephrotic syndrome *KidneyInt*. 1989; 36(Suppl 27):S152–S153.

Pastors JG. Nutrition assessment for diabetes medical nutrition therapy. *DiabetesSpectrum*. 1996; 9(2):99–103,

Rabelink TJ, Stroes ESG, Koomans HA. Mechanisms of cardiovascular injury in renal disease. *BloodPurif*. 1996; 14:67–74.

Ruilope LM, Campo C, Rodicio. Blood pressure control, proteinuria and renal outcome in chronic renal failure. *CurrOpinNephrolHypertens*. 1998; 7:145–148.

Schneeweiss R, Graninger W, Stockenhuber F, et al. Energy metabolism in acute and chronic renal failure. *AmJClinNutr*. 1990; 52:596–601.

Scopelite JA. Dietary modifications: Impact on diabetic nephropathy. *ANNAJ*. 1992; 1 19(5):447–452.

Silverman M, Bakris GL. Treatment of renal failure and blood pressure. *CurrOpinNephrolHypertension*. 1997; 6:237–242.

Stover J (ed). *A Clinical Guide to Nutrition Care in End-Stage Renal Disease* (2nd ed). Chicago, Ill: American Dietetic Association; 1994.

Sunder-Plassmann G, Horl WH. Erythropoietin and iron. *ClinNephrol*. 1997; 47(3):141–157.

Tsukamoto Y, Moriya R, Nagaba Y, Morishita T, Izumida I, Okubu M. Effect of administering calcium carbonate to treat secondary hyperparathyroidism in nondialyzed patients with chronic renal failure. *AmJKidneyDis*. 1995; 25(6):879–886.

Wenger NK. Lipid metabolism, physical activity, and postmenopausal hormone therapy. *AmJKidneyDis*. 1998; 32(5,Suppl 3):S80–S88.

Wheeler DC. Cardiovascular risk factors in patients with chronic renal failure. *JRenalNutr*. 1997; 7(4):182–186 .

Yamamoto ME, Olson MB, Fine J, Powers S, Stollar C. The effect of sodium restriction and weight reduction on blood pressure of patients with hypertension and chronic renal disease. *JRenalNutr*. 1997; 7(1):25–32.

Guideline 2
Nutrition Care of Adult Dialysis Patients

Synopsis/Summary

Diagnosis: End-Stage Renal Disease (Adult 18+ years)

Treatment Mode: Hemodialysis or Peritoneal Dialysis

Setting: Outpatient Dialysis Center or Home Dialysis

Exceptions for Chart Audit: Patients who are younger than 18 years of age; patients who transfer to another unit, receive transplants, or die within 1 month; patients visiting from another unit for less than 2 months. For subjective data, patients who are unwilling or unable to communicate and have no caregivers who wish to do so.

Encounter*	Length of Contact	Intervals Between Encounters
Initial	60–90 minutes	Within 1 month of admission or initiation of dialysis
Follow-up	30–45 minutes	1 month
Nutritional Updates	45–60 minutes	Every 6 months and as indicated

* In-center hemodialysis patients are routinely followed by the dialysis facility's renal dietitian with counseling and interventions provided on an ongoing basis. Laboratory values and patient status are typically monitored on a monthly basis with interventions made in response to aberrant labs. Comprehensive nutritional assessments are performed yearly.

End-Stage Renal Disease, Dialysis Flowchart

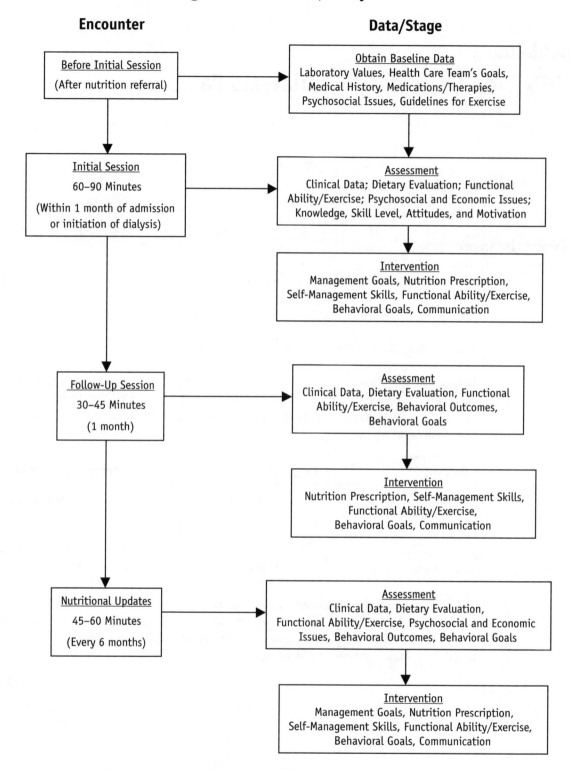

Encounter

Data/Stage

Before Initial Session
(After nutrition referral)

Obtain Baseline Data
Laboratory Values, Health Care Team's Goals,
Medical History, Medications/Therapies,
Psychosocial Issues, Guidelines for Exercise

Initial Session
60–90 Minutes
(Within 1 month of admission
or initiation of dialysis)

Assessment
Clinical Data; Dietary Evaluation; Functional
Ability/Exercise; Psychosocial and Economic Issues;
Knowledge, Skill Level, Attitudes, and Motivation

Intervention
Management Goals, Nutrition Prescription,
Self-Management Skills, Functional Ability/Exercise,
Behavioral Goals, Communication

Follow-Up Session
30–45 Minutes
(1 month)

Assessment
Clinical Data, Dietary Evaluation, Functional
Ability/Exercise, Behavioral Outcomes,
Behavioral Goals

Intervention
Nutrition Prescription, Self-Management Skills,
Functional Ability/Exercise,
Behavioral Goals, Communication

Nutritional Updates
45–60 Minutes
(Every 6 months)

Assessment
Clinical Data, Dietary Evaluation,
Functional Ability/Exercise, Psychosocial and Economic
Issues, Behavioral Outcomes, Behavioral Goals

Intervention
Management Goals, Nutrition Prescription,
Self-Management Skills, Functional Ability/Exercise,
Behavioral Goals, Communication

Expected Outcomes of Medical Nutrition Therapy

Outcome Assessment Factors	Expected Outcome of Therapy	Ideal/Goal Value
Clinical Outcomes • Biochemical Parameters —BUN, creatinine —Albumin —Potassium —Phosphorus —Calcium —Serum glucose (casual) —HbA1c (diabetes) —Cholesterol —PTH (intact) • Hematological Parameters —Hematocrit/hemoglobin —Ferritin —Transferrin saturation • Dialysis Adequacy —Kt/V (URR) —nPNA (stable state) • Anthropometrics —Dry weight —Interdialytic fluid gains (Hemodialysis) • Clinical Signs and Symptoms	**Measure < 30 days prior to nutrition session** —BUN and creatinine levels stabilized —Albumin increasing to ≥ 4.0 —Potassium maintained within goal range —Phosphorus and calcium levels progressing toward goal ranges —Blood sugar levels maintained within goal range —Cholesterol levels progressing toward goal range —PTH maintained within goal range —Adequate erythropoiesis maintained —Adequate iron stores maintained for erythropoiesis —Kt/V (URR) maintained at or above target goal —nPNA maintained at or above goal —Reasonable weight achieved/ maintained —Fluid gains achieved/maintained at goal —Adequate body mass maintained —Level of functional ability maintained —Good appetite maintained —Appropriate blood pressure control maintained	 —BUN and creatinine levels stabilized —Albumin ≥ 4.0 g/dL —Potassium 3.5–5.5 mEq/L —Phosphorus 4.0–6.0 mg/dL —Calcium 8.5–10.5 mg/dL —Serum glucose 80–200 mg/dL —HbA1c < 7% —Cholesterol 150–250 mg/dL —PTH 100–300 pg/mL —Hematocrit 33–36%, hemoglobin 11.0–12.0 g/dL —Ferritin 100–800 ng/mL —Transferrin saturation 20%–50% —Kt/V ≥ 1.2 or URR 65 (hemodialysis) —Weekly Kt/V ≥ 2.0, creatinine clearance ≥ 60 liters/wk/1.73 m² (CAPD) —nPNA ≥ 0.8 —Within reasonable body weight (BMI 20–25) —Fluid gains 2–5% body weight —Adequate muscle/fat stores —Optimum functional ability —Minimum GI symptoms —Food intake > 80% recommended intake —Blood pressure within appropriate limits
Patient/Caregiver Behavioral Outcomes • Food selection/meal planning • Nutrient needs • Potential food/drug interactions • Exercise	 —Exhibits positive changes in food selection and amounts —If diabetic, times meals and snacks appropriately —Identifies foods high in protein, sodium, potassium, and phosphorus content —Identifies fluid sources and limits —Verbalizes potential food/drug interactions —If no medical limitations, gradually increases or continues physical activity level	**MNT Goals** 1. Makes appropriate food choices and takes medications as prescribed. 2. Maintains adequate protein intake 3. Maintains lab values within acceptable limits 4. If diabetic, maintains stable glucose levels through appropriate dietary practices. 5. If no medical limitations, maintenance of an exercise program

Minimum Baseline Data Needed for Medical Nutrition Therapy

Factor	Data Needed
Laboratory Values with Dates (within 30 days of session)	1. BUN, creatinine 2. Albumin 3. Sodium, potassium, phosphorus, calcium 4. Serum glucose 5. Serum bicarbonate 6. PTH, if available 7. Hematocrit/hemoglobin 8. Ferritin, transferrin saturation 9. Dialysis adequacy and PET results 10. Urinalysis results (e.g., volume, urea, protein) 11. Others as appropriate (e.g., lipid profile, glycosylated hemoglobin, vitamin B12, folate)
Health Care Team's Goals for Patient	1. Patient prognosis 2. Expected outcome of nutrition therapy 3. Aggressive versus conservative measures
Medical History	1. Disease/condition causing *Renal Failure* 2. History of renal disease and treatment 3. Concurrent medical conditions (e.g., diabetes, cancer, HIV, cardiovascular disease, GI problems, hypertension, hyperlipidemia) 4. Any other medical or physical coditions with potential nutritional implications (e.g., surgery, infection, CVA, chemotherapy, blindness, neuropathies)
Medications/Therapies	1. Type of dialysis therapy and prescription 2. Diet order, tube-feeding order, parenteral nutrition order, and/or IDPN/IPN order 3. Any other treatments or therapies that may affect nutritional intake or status 4. Antihypertensives, diuretics 5. Anticoagulants 6. Phosphate binders 7. Vitamin/mineral supplements 8. Any other medications with food/drug interactions or nutritional impact (e.g., diabetes medications, GI medications, steroids)
Psychosocial Issues	1. Learning disabilities 2. Vision, hearing abilities 3. Cultural or language barriers 4. Mental status
Guidelines for Exercise	1. Medical clearance for exercise 2. Exercise limitations, if any

Initial Nutrition Assessment

Session: *Initial*   Length: *60–90 minutes*   Time: *Within 1 month of admission or dialysis initiation*

Factor	Assessments
Clinical Data	1. Review Minimum Baseline Data table. 2. Obtain current height, dry weight, and BMI. 3. Obtain weight history, recent weight changes, and weight goals. 4. Determine IBW and/or UBW adjusted for amputation or obesity, and percentage IBW and/or percentage UBW (see Appendix B). 5. Assess muscle and fat stores, presence of edema. 6. Assess for physical signs of nutrient deficiencies/excesses or increased needs (e.g., decubiti, poor wound healing, thinning hair, pale conjunctiva, cheilosis). 7. Determine nitrogen balance using urea kinetics, if appropriate (see Appendix D). 8. Assess blood pressure control.
Dietary Evaluation	1. Determine previous dietary instruction and practices. 2. Determine usual food intake and pattern of intake. 3. Assess appetite, GI issues, tolerance of oral intake, and food allergies/intolerances. 4. Assess feeding issues (e.g., chewing, swallowing). 5. Determine use of vitamin/mineral, herbal, or other nutrition supplements. 6. Determine alcohol/drug/tobacco use and history. 7. For PD, determine glucose absorption and calories from dialysate (see Appendix C). 8. Assess intake of calories, protein, sodium, potassium, phosphorus, calcium, fluids, and other nutrients as indicated. 9. Assess diet order, tube-feeding order, parenteral nutrition order, and/or IDPN/IPN order for appropriateness.
Functional Ability/Exercise	1. Determine level of functional ability and recent changes. 2. Assess ability to feed self and needs for assistance. 3. Determine activity level and exercise habits. 4. Determine physical or motivational limitations to exercise.
Psychosocial and Economic Issues	1. Assess living situation, cooking facilities, finances, educational background, employment, literacy, and other factors that may affect availability of food. 2. Assess ethnic or religious belief considerations. 3. Assess availability of support systems. 4. Determine whether other relevant psychosocial or economic issues exist.
Knowledge, Skill Level, Attitudes, and Motivation	1. Assess basic knowledge level of dietary guidelines for patient's mode of treatment. 2. Assess basic knowledge level of impact of renal disease on nutrition. 3. Assess attitudes toward nutrition and health. 4. Determine patient's willingness and ability to learn and make appropriate changes.

Initial Nutrition Intervention

Session: *Initial*   **Length:** *60–90 minutes*   **Time:** *Within 1 month of admission or dialysis initiation*

Factor	Interventions
Management Goals	1. Identify management goals of health care team. 2. Identify patient goals and expectations.
Nutrition Prescription	1. Calories—individualized; use basal energy expenditure × activity factor (1.2–1.3) × stress factor; or use 30–35 kcal/kg IBW or adjusted weight (hemodialysis); 25–35 kcal/kg IBW or adjusted weight (peritoneal dialysis-includes calories from dialysate glucose absorption) 2. Protein = 1.1–1.4 g/kg IBW or adjusted weight (hemodialysis); 1.2–1.5 g/kg IBW or adjusted weight (peritoneal dialysis); may be higher depending on stress or metabolic needs 3. Fats—for lipid abnormalities: fats, cholesterol, and carbohydrates adjusted per severity of risk factors (see Appendixes G and H) 4. Sodium—individualized, approximately 2–3 g/day (hemodialysis); 2–4 g/day (peritoneal dialysis) 5. Potassium—individualized, approximately. 40 mg/kg IBW or adjusted weight (hemodialysis); restricted only by lab values (peritoneal dialysis) 6. Phosphorus—individualized, approximately ≤ 17 mg/kg IBW or adjusted weight; may require phosphate binder therapy 7. Calcium—individualized per calcium, phosphorus, and PTH lab values and use of vitamin D; approximately 1000–1500 mg/day 8. Fluids—500–750 mL + urine output per day (or 1000 mL/day if anuric) (hemodialysis); to maintain fluid balance (peritoneal dialysis) 9. Vitamin/mineral supplementation—as appropriate
Self-Management Skills	1. Discuss simple definitions and examples of calories, protein, and other nutrients as is appropriate (e.g., fats, sodium, potassium, phosphorus, calcium, fluids). 2. Discuss basic dietary guidelines for ESRD. 3. For diabetes, discuss basic dietary guidelines and timing of meals and snacks, if indicated. 4. Discuss dry weight and fluid restrictions if appropriate. 5. Discuss laboratory tests and significance of results. 6. Discuss use and effect of phosphate binders. 7. Discuss food/drug interactions as indicated. 8. Discuss role and effect of diet and medications on renal disease and dialysis treatment. 9. Assess comprehension of education provided and projected compliance.
Functional Ability/Exercise	1. Provide necessary referrals for assistance with self-feeding and other activities of daily living (e.g., OT, PT, speech therapy). 2. Discuss exercise recommendations, if appropriate.
Behavioral Goals	1. Address eating and exercise behaviors. 2. Identify and summarize short-term behavioral goals that are specific and achievable. 3. Establish follow-up plan.
Communication	1. Document current nutritional status, plan of care, and goals of MNT. 2. Report recommendations/concerns to appropriate health care team member (e.g., MD, RN, pharmacist, social worker). 3. Provide information regarding nutrition prescription and dietary guidelines to extended-care facility, home health care facilities, if appropriate.

Follow-up Nutrition Assessment

Session: *Follow-up*   Length: *30–45 minutes*   Time: *1 month*

Factor	Assessments
Clinical Data	1. Review changes in medical status and recent/planned therapies (e.g., medication, dialysis, surgery). 2. Review any new or updated laboratory data. 3. Assess changes in dry weight and interdialytic weight changes, if appropriate. 4. Assess muscle and fat stores, presence of edema. 5. Assess for physical signs of nutrient deficiencies/excesses or increased needs (e.g., decubiti, poor wound healing, thinning hair, pale conjunctiva, cheilosis). 6. Review dialysis adequacy and PET results, if available. 7. Assess blood pressure control. 8. Assess effectiveness of previous nutrition intervention.
Dietary Evaluation	1. Determine current GI or feeding issues or concerns. 2. Assess changes in patient's food intake and/or appetite. 3. For PD, determine glucose absorption and calories from dialysate (see Appendix C). 4. Assess dietary intake and/or nutritional support intake for adequacy and appropriateness.
Functional Ability/Exercise	1. Assess changes in functional ability. 2. Assess changes in activity level or exercise habits.
Behavioral Outcomes	1. Assess understanding of simple definitions and examples of calories, protein, and other nutrients as appropriate (e.g., fats, sodium, potassium, phosphorus, calcium, fluids). 2. Assess understanding of basic dietary guidelines for ESRD. 3. For diabetes, assess understanding of basic dietary guidelines and timing of meals and snacks. 4. Assess understanding of dry weight and fluid restrictions. 5. Assess understanding of laboratory tests and significance of results. 6. Assess understanding of use and effect of phosphate binders. 7. Assess understanding of food/drug interactions. 8. Assess understanding of role and effect of diet and medications on renal disease and dialysis treatment. 9. Determine further improvements that can be made in the quality of the diet.
Behavioral Goals	1. Assess achievement of prior behavioral goals. 2. Determine willingness and ability to make further changes.

Follow-up Nutrition Intervention

Session: *Follow-up*   Length: *30–45 minutes*   Time: *1 month*

Factor	Interventions
Nutrition Prescription	1. Provide feedback on lab results, blood pressure control, changes in weight. 2. Provide feedback on food/meal plan, food choices and portions. 3. Recommend changes in nutrient intake or habits that may improve outcomes. 4. Adjust MNT as is appropriate.
Self-Management Skills	1. Review and reinforce self-management skills from first session. 2. Provide and review educational materials as is appropriate. 3. If medication change, discuss potential food/drug interaction. 4. Assess comprehension of education provided and projected compliance.
Functional Ability/Exercise	1. Refer to OT, PT, speech therapy as is appropriate. 2. Discuss changes in exercise recommendations, if appropriate.
Behavioral Goals	1. Reset short-term behavioral goals that are specific and achievable. 2. Review and reinforce long-term goals. 3. Establish follow-up plan.
Communication	1. Document current nutritional status, plan of care, and goals of MNT. 2. Report recommendations/concerns to appropriate health care team member (e.g., MD, RN, pharmacist, social worker). 3. Provide information regarding nutrition prescription and dietary guidelines to extended-care facility, home health care facilities, if appropriate.

Six-Month Nutrition Assessment

Session: *Nutritional Update*   Length: *45–60 minutes*   Time: *Every 6 months and as indicated*

Factor	Assessments
Clinical Data	1. Review changes in medical status and recent/planned therapies (e.g., medication, dialysis, surgery). 2. Review recent laboratory data. 3. Assess changes in dry weight and interdialytic weight changes, if appropriate. 4. Determine BMI, IBW and/or UBW adjusted for amputation or obesity, and percentage IBW and/or percentage UBW (see Appendix B). 5. Assess muscle and fat stores, presence of edema. 6. Assess for physical signs of nutrient deficiencies/excesses or increased needs (e.g., decubiti, poor wound healing, thinning hair, pale conjunctiva, cheilosis). 7. Review dialysis adequacy and PET results. 8. Determine nitrogen balance using urea kinetics (see Appendix D). 9. Assess blood pressure control. 10. Assess effectiveness of previous nutrition intervention.
Dietary Evaluation	1. Determine current GI or feeding issues or concerns, tolerance of oral intake. 2. Assess changes in patient's food intake and/or appetite. 3. Determine use of vitamin/mineral, herbal, or other nutrition supplements. 4. For PD, determine glucose absorption and calories from dialysate (see Appendix C). 5. Assess intake of calories, protein, sodium, potassium, phosphorus, calcium, fluid, and other nutrients as indicated. 6. Assess diet order, tube-feeding order, parenteral nutrition order, and/or IDPN/IPN order for appropriateness.
Functional Ability/Exercise	1. Determine level of functional ability and recent changes. 2. Assess ability to feed self and needs for assistance. 3. Assess changes in activity level or exercise habits. 4. Determine physical or motivational limitations to exercise.
Psychosocial and Economic Issues	1. Assess changes in living situation, cooking facilities, finances, education, employment, literacy, and other factors that may affect availability of food. 2. Assess availability of support systems. 3. Determine whether other relevant psychosocial or economic issues exist.
Behavioral Outcomes	1. Assess understanding of prior nutrition education and food/meal plan. 2. Assess appropriateness of food intake and pattern of intake. 3. Assess understanding of relevant food/drug interactions. 4. Determine further improvements that can be made in the quality of the diet.
Behavioral Goals	1. Assess achievement of prior behavioral goals. 2. Determine willingness and ability to make further changes.

Six-Month Nutrition Intervention

Session: *Nutritional Update*   Length: *45–60 minutes*   Time: *Every 6 months and as indicated*

Factor	Interventions
Management Goals	1. Reassess and adjust management goals of patient and health care team.
Nutrition Prescription	1. Provide feedback on lab results, blood pressure control, and changes in weight. 2. Provide feedback on food/meal plan, food choices, and portions. 3. Recommend changes in nutrient intake or habits that may improve outcomes. 4. Adjust MNT as appropriate.
Self-Management Skills	1. Review and reinforce self-management skills. 2. Provide and review educational materials as is appropriate. 3. If medication change, discuss potential food/drug interaction. 4. Assess comprehension of education provided and projected compliance.
Functional Ability/Exercise	1. Provide necessary referrals for assistance with self-feeding and other activities of daily living (e.g., OT, PT, speech therapy). 2. Discuss changes in exercise recommendations, if appropriate.
Behavioral Goals	1. Reset short-term behavioral goals that are specific and achievable. 2. Review and reinforce long-term goals. 3. Establish follow-up plan.
Communication	1. Document current nutritional status, plan of care, and goals of MNT. 2. Report recommendations/concerns to appropriate health care team member (e.g., MD, RN, pharmacist, social worker). 3. Provide information regarding nutrition prescription and dietary guidelines to extended-care facility, home health care facilities, if appropriate.

Bibliography

American Diabetes Association Position Statement: Hospital admission guidelines for diabetes mellitus. *Diabetes Care.* 1997;20(Suppl 1):S52.

American Diabetes Association Position Statement: Nutrition Recommendations and Principles for People with Diabetes Mellitus. *Diabetes Care.*1997;20(Suppl 1):S14–S17.

American Diabetes Association Position Statement: Screening for Diabetes. *Diabetes Care.* 1997; 20(Suppl 1):S22–S23.

American Diabetes Association Position Statement: Standards of Medical Care for Patients with Diabetes Mellitus. *Diabetes Care.* 1997;20(Suppl 1):S5–S13.

American Diabetes Association. *Maximizing the Role of Nutrition in Diabetes Management.* Alexandria, Va: American Diabetes Association, Inc; 1994.

Anastassiades EG, Howarth D, Howarth J, Shanks D, Waters HM, Hyde K, Geary CG, Liu Yin JA, Gokal R. Monitoring of iron requirements in renal patients on erythropoietin. *Nephrol Dial Transplant.* 1993;8:846–853.

Andress DL. Treatment of low turnover bone disease in renal failure. *Nephrol Exchange.* 1996;6(1): 16–20.

Antonsen JE, Sherrard DJ. Renal osteodystrophy. *Dial & Transplant.* October 1996:716–719.

Attman PO, Alaupovic P. Lipid Abnormalities in chronic renal insufficiency. *Kidney Int.* 1991;39 (Suppl 31):S16–S23.

Avram MM, Goldwasser P, Erroa M, Fein PA. Predictors of survival in continuous ambulatory peritoneal dialysis patients: The importance of prealbumin and other nutritional and metabolic markers. *Am J Kidney Dis.* 1994;23(1):91–98.

Avram MM, Mittman N, Bonomini L, Chattopadhyay J, Fein P. Markers for survival in dialysis: A seven-year prospective study. *Am J Kidney Dis.* 1995;26(1):209–219.

Avram MM, Sreedhara R, Avram DK, Muchnick RA, Fein P. Enrollment parathyroid hormone level is a new marker of survival in hemodialysis and peritoneal dialysis therapy for uremia. *Am J Kidney Dis.* 1996;28(6):924–930.

Avram MM, Sreedhara R, Mittman N. Long-term survival in end-stage renal disease. *Dial & Transplant* 1998;27(1):11–24.

Bailey JL, Mitch WE. The implications of metabolic acidosis in intensive care unit patients. *Nephrol Dial Transplant.* 1998;13:837–839.

Bargman JM. The rationale and ultimate limitations of urea kinetic modelling in the estimation of nutritional status. *Peritoneal Dial Int.* 1996;16:347–351.

Bergström J, Lindholm B. Nutrition and adequacy of dialysis. How do hemodialysis and CAPD compare? *Kidney Int.* 1993;43(Suppl 40):S39–S50.

Bergström J, Wang T, Lindholm B. Factors contributing to catabolism in end-stage renal disease patients. *Miner Electrolyte Metab.* 1998;24:92–101.

Bergström J. Nutrition and adequacy of dialysis in hemodialysis patients. *Kidney Int.* 1993;43(Suppl 41):S261–S267.

Bergström J. Factors causing catabolism in maintainance hemodialysis patients. *Miner Electrolyte Metab.* 1992;18:280–283.

Beto JA. Which diet for which *Renal Failure.* Making sense of the options. *J Am Diet Assoc.* 1995;95(8):898–903.

Blake PG. Malnutrition in peritoneal dialysis–Part 1. *Contemp Dial & Nephrol.* July 1994:24–26, 34.

Block GA, Hulbert-Shearon TE, Levin NW, Port FK. Association of serum phosphorus and calcium x phosphate product with mortality risk in chronic hemodialysis patients: A national study. *Am J Kidney Dis.* 1998;31(4):607–617.

Bodner DM, Busch S, Fuchs J, Piedmonte M, Schreiber M. Estimating glucose absorption in peritonealdialysis using peritoneal equilibration tests. *Adv Peritoneal Dial.* 1993;9:114–118.

Bourke E, Delaney V. Assessment of hypocalcemia and hypercalcemia. *Clin Lab Med.* 1993; 13(1):157–181.

Brandes JC, Piering WF, Beres JA, Blumenthal SS, Fritsche C. Clinical outcome of continuous ambulatory peritoneal dialysis predicted by urea and creatinine kinetics. *J Am Soc Nephrol.* 1992;2:1430–1435.

Burkart JM. Clinical recommendations of an Ad Hoc Committee on Peritoneal Dialysis Adequacy. *Dial & Transplant.* 1997;26(2):91–95.

Cappuccio FP, MacGregor GA. Dietary salt restriction: benefits for cardiovascular disease and beyond. *Curr Opin Nephrol Hypertens.* 1997;6:477–482.

Castaneda C, Grossi L, Dwyer J. Potential benefits of resistance exercise training on nutritional status in renal failure. *J Renal Nutr.* 1998 Jan;8(1):2–10.

Castaneda C. The relationship between rehabilitation and nutrition status in renal disease patients. *Contemp Dial & Neph.* August 1997:18–21.

Chazan JA, London MR, Pono L. Markedly elevated BUN is not correlated with increased morbidity and mortality in a large chronic hemodialysis population. *Dial & Transplant.* 1991;20(9):547–550.

Cheng IKP, Cy C, Chan MK, Yu L, Fang GX, Wei D. Correction of anemia in patients on continuous ambulatory peritoneal dialysis with subcutaneous recombinant erythropoietin twice a week: A long-term study. *Clinical Nephrol.* 1991;35(5):207–212.

Chertow GM, Bullard A, Lazarus JM. Nutrition and the dialysis prescription. *Am J Nephrol.* 1996;16:79–89.

The Chicago Dietetic Association and The South Suburban Dietetic Association. *Manual of Clinical Dietetics.* 5th ed. Chicago, Ill: The American Dietetic Association; 1996.

Churchill DN. Adequacy of peritoneal dialysis: How much dialysis do we need? *Kidney Int.* 1994;46(Suppl 48):S2–S6.

Coburn JW. Mineral metabolism and renal bone disease: Effects of CAPD versus hemodialysis. *Kidney Int.* 1993;43(Suppl 40):S92–S100.

Cressman MD, Hoogwerf BJ, Schreiber MJ, Cosentino FA. Lipid abnormalities and end-stage renal disease: Implications for atherosclerotic cardiovascular disease? *Miner Electrolyte Metab.* 1993;19:180–185.

Daugirdas JT, Ing TS. *Handbook of Dialysis.* 2nd ed. Boston, Mass: Little, Brown; 1994.

Daview SJ, Russell L, Bryan J, Phillips L, Russell GI. Impact of peritoneal absorption of glucose on appetite, protein catabolism and survival in CAPD patients. *Clin Nephrol.* 1996;45(3):194–198.

Delmez JA, Slatopolsky E. Hyperphosphatemia: Its consequences and treatment in patients with chronic renal disease. *Am J Kidney Dis.* 1992;19(4):303–317.

DeOreo PB. Treatment of anemia of chronic renal failure. *Dial & Transplant.* 1997;26(12):842–844.

Devine W, DiChiro J. Current nutrition management of patients with renal disease. *Top Clin Nutr.* 1992;7(4):21–33.

Dureke TB, Barany P, Cazzola M, Eschbach W, Grutzmacher P, Kaltwasser JP, Macdougall IC, Pippard MJ, Shaldon S, van Wyck D. Management of iron deficiency in renal anemia: Guidelines for the optimal therapeutic approach in erythropoietin-treated patients. *Clin Nephrol.* 1997;48(1):1–8.

Dwyer JT, Cunniff PJ, Maroni BJ, Kopple JD, Burrowes JD, Powers SN, Cockram DB, Chumlea WC, Kusek JW, Makoff R, Goldstein DJ, Paranandi L. The hemodialysis pilot study: Nutrition program and participant characteristics at baseline. *J Renal Nutr.* 1998;8(1):11–20.

Farkas-Hirsch R (ed). *Intensive Diabetes Management.* Alexandria, Va: American Diabetes Association; 1995.

Fishbane S, Maesaka JK. Iron management in end-stage renal disease. *Am J Kidney Dis.* 1997;29(3): 319–333.

Foulks CJ. Nutritional evaluation of patients on maintenance dialysis therapy. *ANNA J.* 1988;15(1): 13–17, 46.

Franco PA. Five markers to help identify malnutrition. *Nephrol News & Issues.* November 1996:21, 64.

Frazao JM, Levine BS, Tan AU, Mazess RB, Kyllo DM, Knutson JC, Bishop CW, Coburn JW. Efficacy and safety of intermittent oral 1-alpha-(OH)-vitamin D2 in suppressing secondary hyperparathyroidism in hemodialysis patients. *Dial & Transplant.* 1997;26(9):583–586, 590–595, 630.

Fung L, Pollock CA, Caterson RJ, Mahony JF, Waugh DA, Macadam C, Ibels LS. Dialysis adequacy and nutrition determine prognosis in continuous ambulatory peritoneal dialysis patients. *J Am Soc Nephrol.* 1996;7:737–744.

Geraghty ME, Cockram DB. Protein-calorie malnutrition in dialysis patients. *Contemp Dial & Nephrol.* November 1991:64, 67–68., 70.

Golder R, Delmez JA, Klahr S. Bone disease in long-term dialysis. *Am J Kidney Dis.* 1996;28(6): 918–923.

Goldstein DJ, Frederico CB. The effect of urea kinetic modeling on the nutrition management of hemodialysis patients. *J Am Diet Assoc.* 1987;87(4):474–479.

Goldwasser P, Mittman N, Antignani A, Burrell D, Michel MA, Collier J, Avram MM. Predictors of mortality in hemodialysis patients. *J Am Soc Nephrol.* 1993;3:1613–1622.

Grant A, DeHoog S. *Nutritional Assessment and Support.* 4th ed. Seattle, Wash: Anne Grant/Susan DeHoog; 1991.

Hakim RM, Levin N. Malnutrition in hemodialysis patients. *Am J Kidney Dis.* 1993;21(2):125–137.

Harty J, Gokal R. Nutritional status in peritoneal dialysis. *J. Renal Nutr.* 1995;5(1):2–10.

Harty J, Venning M, Gokal R. Does CAPD guarantee adequate dialysis delivery and nutrition. *Nephrol Dial Transplant.* 1994;9:1721–1723.

Harty JC, Goldsmith DJA, Boulton H, Heelis N, Uttley L, Morris J, Venning MC, Gokal R. Limitations of the peritoneal equilibration test in prescribing and monitoring dialysis therapy. *Nephrol Dial Transplant.* 1995;10:252–257.

Harum P. Vitamin, mineral, and hormone interactions in renal bone disease. *J Renal Nutr.* 1993;3(1):30–35.

Heimburger O, Bergstrom J, Lindholm B. Maintenance of optimal nutrition in CAPD. *Kidney Int.* 1994;46(Suppl 48):S39–S46.

Heimburger O. Residual renal function, peritoneal transport characteristics and dialysis adequacy in peritoneal dialysis. *Kidney Int.* 1996;50(Suppl 56):S47–S55.

Heimburger O. Residual renal function, peritoneal transport characteristics and dialysis adequacy in peritoneal dialysis. *Kidney Int.* 1996;50(Suppl 56):S47–S55.

Hill LJ, Biesecker RL. Iron supplementation in dialysis patients with regard to cardiovascular disease and iron overload. *Top Clin Nutr.* 1996;12(1):41–50.

Hirschberg RR, Kopple JD. Energy requirements in patients with *Renal Failure.. Contrib Nephrol.* 1990;81:124–135.

Horl WH, Dreyling K, Steinhauer HB, Engelhardt R, Schollmeyer P. Iron status of dialysis patients under rhuEPO therapy. *Contrib Nephrol.* 1990;87:78–86.

Humphries JE. Anemia of *Renal Failure.*: Use of erythropoietin. *Med Clin N Amer.* 1992;76(3):711–725.

Ikizler TA, Wingard RL, Hakim RM. Interventions to treat malnutrition in dialysis patients: The role of the dose of dialysis, intradialytic parenteral nutrition, and growth hormone. *Am J Kidney Dis*. 1995;26(1):256–265.

Ikizler TA, Wingard RL, Sun M, Harvell J, Parker RA, Hakim RM. Increased energy expenditure in hemodialysis patients. *J Am Soc Nephrol*. 1996;7(12):2646–2653.

Ikizler TA. Biochemical markers: Clinical aspects. *J Renal Nutr*. 1997;7(2):61–64.

Iseki K, Kawazoe N, Fukiyama K. Serum albumin is a strong predictor of death in chronic dialysis patients. *Kidney Int*. 1993;44:115–119.

Jacobs L, Rubens-Kenler S, Dwyer J. Evolution of the renal diet in hemodialysis using urea kinetic modeling. *Top Clin Nutr*. 1996;12(1):6–17.

Kaminski MV, Lowrie EG, Rosenblatt SG, Haase T. Malnutrition is lethal, diagnosable, and treatable in ESRD patients. *Transplant Proc*. 1991;23(2):1810–1815.

Karalis M. Malnutrition in the hemodialysis patient. *Renal Nutr Forum*. 1995;14(4):1–4.

Kasiske BL. Hyperlipidemia in patients with chronic renal disease. *Am J Kidney Dis*. 1998;32(5, Suppl 3):S142–S156.

Kaysen GA. Hyperlipidemia of chronic renal failure. *Blood Purif*. 1994;12:60–67.

Kent PS. Nutrition management of diabetes in the adult peritoneal dialysis patient. *Renal Nutr Forum*. 1996;16(4):1–3,18.

Keshaviah P. Urea kinetic and middle molecule approaches to assessing the adequacy of hemodialysis and CAPD. *Kidney Int*. 1993;43(Suppl 40):S28–S38.

Kopple JD. Dietary protein and energy requirements in ESRD patients. *Am J Kidney Dis*. 1998;32(6, Suppl 4):S97–S104.

Kopple JD. Effect of nutrition on morbidity and mortality in maintenance dialysis patients. *Am J Kidney Dis*. 1994;24(6):1002–1009.

Kopple JD, Hakim RM, Held PJ, Keane WF, King K, Lazarus JM, Parker TF, Teehan BP. Recommendations for reducing the high morbidity and mortality of united states maintenance dialysis patients. *Am J Kidney Dis*. 1994;24(6):968–973.

Kopple JD, Massry SG (eds). *Nutritional Management of Renal Disease*. Baltimore, Md: Williams & Wilkins; 1997.

Korbet SM. Anemia and erythropoietin in hemodialysis and continuous ambulatory peritoneal dialysis. *Kidney Int*. 1993;43(40):S111–S119.

Korkor A, Blanchard M. Renal osteodystrophy management with CQI techniques. *Nephrol Exchange*. 1996;6(1):10–15.

Krediet RT, Koomen GCM, Struijk DG, Van Olden RW, Imholz ALT, Boeschoten EW. Practical methods for assessing dialysis efficiency during peritoneal dialysis. *Kidney Int*. 1994;46(Suppl 48):S7–S13.

Lameire N, Bernaert P, Lambert MC, Vijt D. Cardiovascular risk factors and their mangement in patients on continuous ambulatory peritoneal dialysis *Kidney Int*. 1994;46(Suppl 48):S31–S38.

Leavey SF, Strawderman RL, Jones CA, Port FK, Held PJ. Simple nutritional indicators as independent predictors of mortality in hemodialysis patients. *Am J Kidney Dis*. 1998;31(6):997–1006.

Lebovitz HE (ed). *Therapy for Diabetes Mellitus and Related Disorders*. 2nd ed. Alexandria, Va: American Diabetes Association, Inc; 1994.

Leehey DJ. Hemodialysis in the diabetic patient with end-stage renal disease. *Renal Failure*. 1994;16(5):547–553.

Levey AS. Controlling the epidemic of cardiovascular disease in chronic renal disease: Where do we start? *Am J Kidney Dis*. 1998;32(5,Suppl 3):S5–S13.

Levine DZ (ed). *Care of the Renal Patient*. 2nd ed. Philadelphia, Pa: WB Saunders Company; 1991.

Liftman C. Iron status in hemodialysis patients. *Renal Nutr Forum*. 1997;16(4):11–12.

Liftman C. Malnutrition in hemodialysis patients. *Renal Nutr Forum.* 1996;16(4):10–11.

Liftman C. Understanding peritoneal dialysis. *Renal Nutr Forum.* 1997;16(1):16–17.

Llach F, Yudd M. The importance of hyperphosphatemia in the severity of hyperparathyroidism and its treatment in patients with chronic renal failure. *Nephrol Dial Transplant.* 1998;13(Suppl 3):57–61.

Llach F. The importance of achieving optimal control of serum phosphorus. *Nephrol Exchange.* 1996;6(1):2–9.

Lowrie EG, Lew NL. Death risk in hemodialysis patients: The predictive value of commonly measured variables and an evaluation of death rate differences between facilities. *Am J Kidney Dis.* 1990;15(5):458–482.

Lowrie EG. Chronic dialysis treatment: Clinical outcome and related processes of care. *Am J Kidney Dis.* 1994;24(2):255–266.

Macdougall IC, Hutton D, Coles GA, Williams JD. The use of erythropoietin in renal failure. *Postgrad Med J.* 1991;67:9–15.

Mailloux LU, Levey AS. Hypertension in patients with chronic renal disease. *Am J Kidney Dis.* 1998; 32(5,Suppl 3):S120–S141.

Makoff R. The importance and use of iron supplementation in uremia. *Nephrol News & Issues.* June 1992:14–19.

Makoff R. The value of calcium carbonate in treating acidosis, phosphate retention, and hypocalcemia. *Nephrol News & Issues.* July 1991:16–19, 32.

Malberti F, Corradi B, Cosci P, Calliada F, Marcelli D, Imbasciati E. Long-term effects of intravenous calcitriol therapy on the control of secondary hyperparathyroidism. *Am J Kidney Dis.* 1996;28(5):704–712.

Malluche HH, Monier-Faugere MC. Uremic bone disease: Current knowledge, controversial issues, and new horizons. *Miner Electrolyte Metab.* 1991;17:281–296.

McCann L (ed). *Pocket Guide to Nutritional Assessment of the Adult Renal Patient.* 2nd ed. New York, National Kidney Foundation; 1998.

McCann L. National Kidney Foundation dialysis outcomes quality initiative: Implications for renal dietitians. *J. Renal Nutr.* 1997;7(1):39–42.

McCann L. *Subjective Global Assessment.* Redwood City, Calif: Satellite Dialysis Centers, Inc; 1997.

McCann L. Subjective global assessment as it pertains to the nutritional status of dialysis patients. *Dial & Transplant.* 1996;25(4):190–199, 202, 225.

McCann L, Yates L, Ezaki-Yamaguchi J, Akiyama P. Forms to monitor and assess nutritional status of renal patients. *J Renal Nutr.* 1995;5(3):151–155.

McCusker FX, Teehan BP, Thorpe KE, Keshaviah PR, Churchill DN. How much peritoneal dialysis is required for the maintenance of a good nutritional state? *Kidney Int.* 1996;50(Suppl 56):S56–S61.

McCusker FX, Teehan BP. Peritoneal dialysis: An evolving understanding. *Semin Nephrol.* 1997;17(3):226–238.

Mendley SR, Majkowski NL, Higgins PK. Estimation of urea and creatinine clearance in peritoneal dialysis. *ASAIO J.* 1992;M373–M376.

Mitch WE. Influence of metabolic acidosis on nutrition. *Am J Kidney Dis.* 1997;29(5):xivi–xiviii.

Mitch WE. Mechanisms causing muscle wasting in uremia. *J Renal Nutr.* 1996;6(2):75–78.

Moore LW. Nutrition implications of the proposed clinical practice guidelines for peritoneal dialysis. *Renal Nutr Forum.* 1997;16(4):1–4.

Morbidity and Mortality of Dialysis. NIH Consensus Statement November 1–3, 1993;11(2):1–33.

Movilli E, Bossini N, Viola BF, Camerini C, Cancarini GC, Feller P, Strada A, Maiorca R. Evidence for an independent role of metabolic acidosis on nutritional status in haemodialysis patients. *Nephrol Dial Transplant.* 1998;13:674–678.

Movilli E, Zani R, Carli O, Sangalli L, Pola A, Camerini C, Cancarini GC, Scolari F, Feller P, Maiorca R. Correction of metabolic acidosis increases serum albumin concentrations and decreases kinetically evaluated protein intake in haemodialysis patients: A prospective study. *Nephrol Dial Transplant.* 1998;13:1719–1722.

Muirhead N, Bargman J, Burgess E, Jindal KK, Levin A, Nolin L, Parfrey P. Evidence-based recommendations for the clinical use of recombinant human erythropoietin. *Am J Kidney Dis.* 1995;26(2,Suppl 1):S1–S24.

Nagao K, Tsuchihashi K, Ura N, Nakata T, Shimamoto K. Appropriate hematocrit levels of erythropoietin supplementary therapy in end-stage *Renal Failure.* complicated by coronary artery disease. *Can J Cardiol.* 1997;13(8):747–753.

Nakai S, Shinzato T, Takai I, Fujita Y, Maeda K. Relationship of protein catabolic rate or Kt/V with morbidity. *ASAIO J.* 1993;M602–M605.

Nissenson AR. Achieving target hematocrit in dialysis patients: New Concepts in Iron Management. *Am J Kidney Dis.* 1997;30(6):907–911.

Nissenson AR. Optimal hematocrit for hemodialysis. *Curr Opin Nephrol Hypertens.* 1997;6:524–527.

Nissenson AR. Anemia management: Critical care for the dialysis patient. *Dial & Transplant.* 1006;25(9):579–585,609.

NKF-DOQI Clinical Practice Guidelines for Hemodialysis Adequacy. New York, NY: National Kidney Foundation; 1997.

NKF-DOQI Clinical Practice Guidelines for Peritoneal Dialysis Adequacy. New York, NY: National Kidney Foundation; 1997.

NKF-DOQI Clinical Practice Guidelines for the Treatment of Anemia of Chronic Renal Failure. New York, NY: National Kidney Foundation; 1997.

Oda H, Keane WF. Lipid abnormalities in end stage renal disease. *Nephrol Dial Transplant.* 1998;13(Suppl 1):45–49.

Oldrizzi L, Rugiu C, Maschio G. Nutrition and the kidney: How to manage patients with renal failure. *Nutr Clin Pract.* 1994;9:3–10.

Outcome Measures in patients with ESRD. *Am J Kidney Dis.* 1999;33(4, Suppl 1):S10–S16.

Owen WF, Lew NL, Liu Y, Lowrie EG, Lazarus JM. The urea reduction ratio and serum albumin concentration as predictors of mortality in patients undergoing hemodialysis. *N Engl J Med.* 1993;329:1001–1006.

Owen WF. Nutrition status and survival in end-stage renal disease patients. *Miner Electrolyte Metab.* 1998;24:72–81.

Park L, Uhthoff T, Tierney M, Nadler S. Effect of an intravenous iron dextran regimen on iron stores, hemoglobin, and erythropoietin requirements in hemodialysis patients. *Am J Kidney Dis.* 1998;31(5):835–840.

Pastors JG. Nutrition assessment for diabetes medical nutrition therapy. *Diabetes Spectrum.* 1996;9(2):99–103.

Pedro-Botet J, Senti M, Rubies-Prat J, Pelegri A, Romero R. When to treat dyslipidemia of patients with chronic *Renal Failure.* on haemodialysis? A need to define specific guidelines. *Nephrol Dial Transplant.* 1996;11:308–313.

Pollock CA, Ibels LS, Allen BJ. Nutritional markers and survival in maintenance dialysis patients. *Nephron.* 1996;74:625–641.

Rabelink TJ, Stroes ESG, Koomans HA. Mechanisms of cardiovascular injury in renal disease. *Blood Purif.* 1996;14:67–74.

Ritz E. Why are lipids not predictive of cardiovascular death in the dialysis patient? *Miner Electrolyte Metab.* 1996;22:9–12.

Russell L, Rowley V, Davies S, Russell G. Maintaining adequate nutrition on dialysis. Nursing standard 1996;10(16):25–28.

Schneeweiss R, Graninger W, Stockenhuber F, Druml W, Ferenci P, Eichinger S, Grimm G, Laggner AN, Lenz K. Energy metabolism in acute and chronic renal failure. *Am J Clin Nutr.* 1990;52:596–601.

Scopelite JA. Dietary modifications: Impact on diabetic nephropathy. *ANNA J.* 1992;19(5):447–452.

Sehgal AR, Leon J, Soinski JA. Barriers to adequate protein nutrition among hemodialysis patients. *J. Renal Nutr.* 1998;8(4):179–187.

Selgas R, Bajo MA, Fernandez-Reyes MJ, Bosque E, Lopez-Revuelta K, Jimenez C, Borrego F, de Alvaro F. An analysis of adequacy of dialysis in a selected population on CAPD for over 3 years: The influence of urea and creatinine kinetics. *Nephrol Dial Transplant.* 1993;8:1244–1253.

Sherman RA, Cody RP, Rogers ME, Solanchick JC. Interdialytic weight gain and nutritional parameters in chronic hemodialysis patients. *Am J Kidney Dis.* 1995;25(4):579–583.

Staab P. Back to Basics: An overview of renal osteodystrophy. *Renal Nutr Forum.* 1994;13(2):6–7.

Staab P. Understanding iron balance in hemodialysis patients. *Renal Nutr Forum.* 1994;13(1):6–7.

Stover J (ed). *A Clinical Guide to Nutrition Care in End-Stage Renal Disease.* 2nd ed. Chicago, Ill: The American Dietetic Association; 1994.

Sunder-Plassmann G, Horl WH. Erythropoietin and iron. *Clin Nephrol.* 1997;47(3):141–157.

Sunder-Plassmann G, Horl WH. Laboratory diagnosis of anaemia in dialysis patients: Use of common laboratory tests. *Curr Opin Nephrol Hypertens.* 1997;6:566–569.

Testa A, Beaud JM. The other side of the coin: Interdialytic weight gain as an index of good nutrition. *Am J Kidney Dis.* 1998;31(5):830–834.

Thomas ME, Moorhead JF. Lipids in CAPD: A review. *Contrib Nephrol.* 1990;85:92–99.

Toto RD. Treatment of dyslipidemia in chronic renal failure. *Blood Purif.* 1996;14:75–82.

Tzamaloukas AH, Murata GH. Adequacy of continuous ambulatory peritoneal dialysis. *Int J Artif Organs.* 1993;16(8):567–572.

Van Wyck DB. Iron management during recombinant human erythropoietin therapy. *Am J Kidney Dis.* 1989;14(2, Suppl 1):9–13.

Walls J, Bennett SE. Maintaining nutrition in CAPD patients. *Contrib Nephrol.* 1990;85:79–83.

Walls J. Effect of correction of acidosis on nutritional status in dialysis patients. *Miner Electrolyte Metab.* 1997;23:234–236.

Wenger NK. Lipid metabolism, physical activity, and postmenopausal hormone therapy. *Am J Kidney Dis.* 1998;32(5,Suppl 3):S80–S88.

Wheeler DC. Cardiovascular risk factors in patients with chronic renal failure. *J Renal Nutr.* 1997;7(4):182–186.

Wish JB, Paganini EP, Stivelman J. *Optimizing Care in ESRD: A Focus on Anemia. Bridging the Gap: Bringing Research to Practice.* New York, NY: Triclinica Communications, Inc; 1995.

York S. Current Perspectives: Iron management during therapy with recombinant human erythropoietin. *ANNA J.* 1993;20(6):645–650.

Zarling EJ, Gottlieb K. Nutrition aspects of continuous ambulatory peritoneal dialysis: A Review. *J Am Coll Nutr.* 1994;13(2):133–138.

Zazra JJ. Biochemical markers of nutrition: Technical aspects. *J Renal Nutr.* 1997;7(2):65–68.

Zucchelli P, Santoro A. Correction of acid-base balance by dialysis. *Kidney Int.* 1993;43(Suppl 41):S179–S183.

Guideline 3

Enteral/Parenteral Nutrition Support of Adult Dialysis Patients

Synopsis/Summary

Diagnosis: End-Stage Renal Disease, Tube-Feeding, or Parenteral Nutrition Support (Adult 18+ years)

Treatment Mode: Hemodialysis or Peritoneal Dialysis

Setting: Outpatient Dialysis Center or Home Dialysis

Exceptions for Chart Audit: Patients who are younger than 18 years of age; patients who transfer to another unit, receive transplants, or die within 1 month; patients visiting from another unit for less than 2 months. For subjective data, patients who are unwilling or unable to communicate and have no caregivers who wish to do so.

Encounter*	Length of Contact	Intervals Between Encounters
Initial	60–90 minutes	Within 72 hours of institution of nutrition support or nutrition referral
Follow-up	30–45 minutes	1–3 times per week for 2 weeks or until stable*
Nutritional Updates	30–45 minutes	Monthly or as indicated

* See Appendix F to determine frequency of monitoring of laboratory and nutritional data.

Acute Renal Failure Flowchart

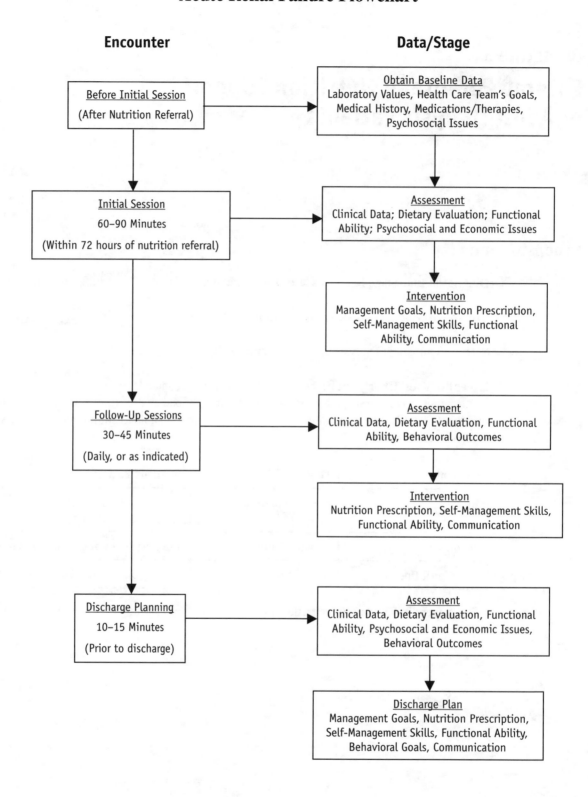

Encounter

Data/Stage

Before Initial Session
(After Nutrition Referral)

Obtain Baseline Data
Laboratory Values, Health Care Team's Goals,
Medical History, Medications/Therapies,
Psychosocial Issues

Initial Session
60–90 Minutes
(Within 72 hours of nutrition referral)

Assessment
Clinical Data; Dietary Evaluation; Functional
Ability; Psychosocial and Economic Issues

Intervention
Management Goals, Nutrition Prescription,
Self-Management Skills, Functional
Ability, Communication

Follow-Up Sessions
30–45 Minutes
(Daily, or as indicated)

Assessment
Clinical Data, Dietary Evaluation, Functional
Ability, Behavioral Outcomes

Intervention
Nutrition Prescription, Self-Management Skills,
Functional Ability, Communication

Discharge Planning
10–15 Minutes
(Prior to discharge)

Assessment
Clinical Data, Dietary Evaluation, Functional
Ability, Psychosocial and Economic Issues,
Behavioral Outcomes

Discharge Plan
Management Goals, Nutrition Prescription,
Self-Management Skills, Functional Ability,
Behavioral Goals, Communication

Expected Outcomes of Medical Nutrition Therapy

Outcome Assessment Factors	Expected Outcome of Therapy	Ideal/Goal Value

Clinical Outcomes
• Biochemical Parameters
  —BUN, creatinine
  —Albumin/prealbumin
 	
  —Sodium
  —Potassium
  —Phosphorus
  —Calcium
  —Magnesium
  —Serum glucose (casual)
 	
  —HbA1c (diabetes)
 	
  —Triglycerides
 	
  —Liver enzymes: SGOT, SGPT, total bilirubin, alkaline phosphatase
  —Chloride
  —CO_2
	—BUN and creatinine levels stabilized
	—Albumin/prealbumin levels stabilized or moving toward goal range
	—Sodium and potassium levels maintained within goal ranges
	—Phosphorus, calcium, magnesium levels maintained within goal ranges
	
	—Blood sugar levels maintained within goal range
	
	—Triglycerides maintained within goal range
	
	—Liver enzymes maintained within goal ranges
	
	—Chloride and CO_2 levels maintained within goal ranges
		—BUN and creatinine levels stabilized
		—Albumin $\geq$ 4.0 g/dL, prealbumin $\geq$ 30 mg/dL
		—Sodium 135–145 mEq/L
		—Potassium 3.5–5.5 mEq/L
		—Phosphorus 2.5–6.0 mg/dL
		—Calcium 8.5–10.5 mg/dL
		—Magnesium 1.5–2.0 mEq/L
		—Serum glucose 80–200 mg/dL (enteral), 150–250 mg/dL (parenteral)
		—HbA1c < 7%
		—Triglycerides < 250 mg/dL 4 hrs after lipids stopped, < 400 mg/dL during continuous infusion
		—Liver enzymes within normal laboratory limits
		
		—Chloride 100–106 mEq/L
		
		—CO_2 24–30 mEq/L

• Hematological Parameters
  —Hematocrit/hemoglobin
 	
  —Ferritin
  —Transferrin saturation
	—Adequate erythropoiesis maintained
	
	—Adequate iron stores maintained for erythropoiesis
		—Hematocrit 33–36% hemoglobin 11.0–12.0 g/dL
		—Ferritin 100–800 ng/mL
		—Transferrin saturation 20–50%

• Dialysis Adequacy
  —Kt/V (URR)
 	
  —nPNA (stable state)
	—Kt/V (URR) maintained at or above target goal
	
	—nPNA maintained at or above goal
		—Kt/V $\geq$ 1.2 or URR 65% (hemodialysis)
		—Weekly Kt/V $\geq$ 2.0, creatinine clearance 60 liters/wk/1.73 m^2 (CAPD)
		—nPNA $\geq$ 0.8

• Anthropometrics
  —Dry weight
 	
  —Interdialytic fluid gains (hemodialysis)
	—Lean body mass preserved
	
	—Fluid gains achieved/maintained at goal
		—Within reasonable body weight (BMI 20–25)
		—Fluid gains 2–5% body weight

• Clinical Signs and Symptoms	—Adequate body mass maintained —Level of functional ability maintained —Good appetite maintained —Appropriate blood pressure control maintained	—Adequate muscle/fat stores —Optimum functional ability —Minimum GI symptoms —Dietary intake > 80% recommended intake —Blood pressure within appropriate limits

Continued

Expected Outcomes of Medical Nutrition Therapy (continued)

Outcome Assessment Factors	Expected Outcome of Therapy	Ideal/Goal Value
Patient/Caregiver Behavioral Outcomes • Proper administration of nutritional support • Formula components and dosage • Safe and sanitary administration practices • Response to complications • Record keeping • Potential food/drug interactions	—Administers nutritional support at proper times and rates and through proper methods —Administers formula according to prescription —Employs safe and sanitary practices in administration of nutritional support —Responds appropriately to complications which may arise —Completes intake/output and formula usage records accurately —Verbalizes potential food/drug interactions	**MNT Goals** 1. Maintains/achieves appropriate weight and protein status 2. Maintains appropriate hydration status 3. Maintains appropriate electrolyte and mineral status 4. Prevents infection 5. Avoids/prevents metabolic, mechanical, or GI complications

Minimum Baseline Data Needed for Medical Nutrition Therapy

Factor	Data Needed
Laboratory Values With Dates	1. BUN, creatinine 2. Albumin/prealbumin 3. Sodium, potassium 4. Phosphorus, calcium, magnesium 5. Serum glucose 6. Triglycerides 7. Liver enzymes (SGOT, SGPT, total bilirubin, alk phos) 8. Chloride, CO_2 9. Hematocrit/hemoglobin 10. Dialysis adequacy and PET results, if available 11. Urinalysis results (e.g., volume, urea, protein) 12. Others as appropriate (e.g., glycosylated hemoglobin, PTH, ferritin)
Health Care Team's Goals for Patient	1. Patient prognosis and expected duration of nutrition support 2. Expected outcome of nutrition therapy 3. Aggressive versus conservative measures
Medical History	1. Disease/condition causing renal failure 2. History of renal disease and treatment 3. Indications for nutritional support (e.g., non-functioning GI tract, inability to obtain adequate oral intake, failure of enteral nutrition trials) 4. Extent of factors affecting food ingestion 5. Concurrent medical conditions (e.g., diabetes, HIV, cardiovascular disease, hypertension, hyperlipidemia) 6. Any other medical or physical conditions with potential nutritional implications (e.g., surgery, infection, CVA, blindness, neuropathies)
Medications/Therapies	1. Type of dialysis therapy and prescription 2. Type and placement of access for nutritional support 3. Diet order, tube-feeding order, parenteral nutrition order, or IDPN/IPN order 4. IV administration 5. Regulation of bowel function 6. Any other therapies/treatments that may affect nutritional intake or status 7. Antihypertensives, diuretics 8. Anticoagulants 9. Phosphate binders 10. Vitamin/mineral supplements 11. Any other medications with food/drug interactions or nutritional impact (e.g., diabetes medications, GI medications, steroids, antibiotics, anticonvulsants)
Psychosocial Issues	1. Learning disabilities 2. Vision, hearing abilities 3. Cultural or language barriers 4. Mental status

Initial Nutrition Assessment

Session: *Initial*   Length: *60–90 minutes*   Time: *Within 72 hours of nutrition referral*

Factor	Assessments
Clinical Data	1. Review Minimum Baseline Data table. 2. Obtain current height, dry weight, and BMI. 3. Obtain weight history, recent weight changes, and weight goals. 4. Determine IBW and/or UBW adjusted for amputation or obesity, and percentage IBW and/or percentage UBW (see Appendix B). 5. Assess muscle and fat stores, presence of edema. 6. Assess for physical signs of nutrient deficiencies/excesses or increased needs (e.g., decubiti, poor wound healing, thinning hair, pale conjunctiva, cheilosis). 7. Determine nitrogen balance using urea kinetics, if appropriate (see Appendix D). 8. Assess blood pressure control.
Dietary Evaluation	1. Determine prior use of enteral or parenteral nutrition support. 2. Determine usual food intake and pattern of intake. 3. Assess history and presence of GI issues (e.g., nausea, vomiting, anorexia, malabsorption, diabetic gastroparesis). 4. Assess feeding issues (e.g., chewing, swallowing). 5. Assess tolerance to oral intake (e.g., allergies, appetite, dysgeusia). 6. Assess bowel function (e.g., diarrhea, constipation, ostomy output). 7. Determine use of vitamin/mineral, herbal, or other nutrition supplements. 8. Determine alcohol/drug/tobacco use and history. 9. For PD, determine glucose absorption and calories from dialysate (see Appendix C). 10. Determine hydration status and assess fluid intake/output. 11. Assess intake of calories, protein, sodium, potassium, phosphorus, calcium, and other nutrients as indicated. 12. Assess diet order, tube-feeding order, parenteral nutrition order, and/or IDPN/IPN order for appropriateness.
Functional Ability	1. Determine level of functional ability and recent changes. 2. Assess ability to feed self and needs for assistance. 3. Determine activity level.
Psychosocial and Economic Issues	1. Assess living situation, cooking facilities, finances, educational background, employment, and literacy, and other factors that may affect availability of food. 2. Assess suitability of home environment for provision of home nutritional support, if indicated. 3. Assess ethnic or religious belief considerations. 4. Assess availability of support systems. 5. Determine if other relevant psychosocial or economic issues exist.
Knowledge, Skill Level, Attitudes, and Motivation	1. Assess basic knowledge level regarding rationale for nutritional support and alternative options. 2. Assess basic knowledge level of impact of nutritional support on nutritional status. 3. Assess patient's and/or caregiver's attitudes toward nutritional support. 4. Determine willingness and ability of patient and/or caregiver to learn nutritional support regimen.

Initial Nutrition Intervention

Session: *Initial*   Length: *60–90 minutes*   Time: *Within 72 hours of nutrition referral*

Factor	Interventions
Management Goals	1. Identify management goals of health care team. 2. Identify patient goals and expectations.
Nutrition Prescription	1. Calories, protein—individualized based on dialysis modality and underlying disease state 2. Sodium, potassium, phosphorus, calcium, magnesium—individualized according to laboratory values and dialysis modality, may need to restrict or supplement 3. Fluids—replace urinary and insensible losses to maintain appropriate hydration status (allow for free water for tube flushing) 4. Vitamin/mineral supplementation—as appropriate and per mode of nutritional support 5. Determine type and formulation of nutrition support therapy (see Appendix E). 6. For enteral nutrition, determine route of administration (e.g., nasogastric, gastrostomy, jejunostomy) and method of administration (e.g., bolus, intermittent, continuous). 7. For parenteral nutrition, determine method of administration (e.g., peripheral/central, TPN/IDPN—see Appendix E). 8. Determine infusion times, infusion rate, and rate of progression, if appropriate.
Self-Management Skills	1. Discuss nutrition therapy with patient and/or caregiver and rationale for nutrition support. 2. Discuss dietary guidelines as indicated. 3. Discuss meal planning, timing of meals and snacks, if appropriate. 4. Discuss timing of insulin, binders, iron, or other medications with feedings, if appropriate. 5. Discuss food/drug interactions as indicated. 6. Discuss identification and/or prevention of possible metabolic, mechanical, or gastrointestinal complications and proper responses to complications. 7. Discuss safe and sanitary techniques for formula storage and administration. 8. Discuss appropriate and accurate methodology for recording formula usage, fluid intake, and fluid output as indicated. 9. Discuss role and effect of nutrition support on nutritional status, renal disease, and dialysis treatment, if appropriate. 10. Assess comprehension of education provided and projected compliance.
Functional Ability	1. Provide necessary referrals for assistance with self-feeding and other activities of daily living (e.g., OT, PT, speech therapy).
Behavioral Goals	1. Identify and summarize short-term behavioral goals that are specific and achievable (e.g weight goals, transition to enteral/oral intake). 2. Establish follow-up plan.
Communication	1. Document current nutritional status, plan of care, and goals of MNT. 2. Report recommendations/concerns to appropriate health care team member (e.g., MD, RN, pharmacist, social worker). 3. Refer to home health agency for home support, if indicated. 4. Provide information regarding nutrition prescription and dietary guidelines to extended-care facility, home health care agencies, if appropriate.

Follow-up Nutrition Assessment

Session: *Follow-up*   Length: *30–45 minutes*   Time: *1–3 times per week for 2 weeks or until stable*

Factor	Assessments
Clinical Data	1. Review changes in medical status and recent/planned therapies (e.g., medications, dialysis, surgery). 2. Review any new or updated laboratory data (see Appendix F). 3. Assess changes in dry weight, interdialytic weight changes if appropriate, and presence of edema. 4. Assess for physical signs of nutrient deficiencies/excesses or increased needs (e.g., decubiti, poor wound healing, thinning hair, pale conjunctiva, cheilosis). 5. Assess blood pressure control. 6. Assess effectiveness of previous nutrition intervention.
Dietary Evaluation	1. Assess tolerance of nutritional support. 2. Determine current GI or feeding issues or concerns. 3. Assess changes in ability to digest, absorb, and tolerate oral intake. 4. Assess bowel function (e.g., diarrhea, constipation, ostomy output). 5. For PD, determine glucose absorption and calories from dialysate (see Appendix C). 6. Determine fluid intake/output and hydration status. 7. Assess dietary intake and/or nutritional support intake for adequacy and appropriateness.
Functional Ability	1. Assess changes in functional ability. 2. Assess changes in activity level.
Behavioral Outcomes	1. Assess understanding of nutrition therapy and rationale for nutrition support. 2. Assess understanding of dietary guidelines. 3. Assess understanding of meal planning, timing of meals and snacks. 4. Assess understanding of timing of insulin, binders, iron, or other medications with feedings. 5. Assess understanding of food/drug interactions. 6. Assess understanding of identification and/or prevention of possible metabolic, mechanical, or gastrointestinal complications and proper responses to complications. 7. Assess understanding of safe and sanitary techniques for formula storage and administration. 8. Assess understanding of appropriate and accurate methodology for recording formula usage, fluid intake, and fluid output as indicated. 9. Assess understanding of role and effect of nutrition support on nutritional status, renal disease and dialysis treatment. 10. Determine further improvements that can be made in administration practices.
Behavioral Goals	1. Assess achievement of prior behavioral goals. 2. Determine willingness and ability to make further changes.

Follow-up Nutrition Intervention

Session: *Follow-up*   Length: *30–45 minutes*   Time: *1–3 times per week for 2 weeks or until stable*

Factor	Interventions
Nutrition Prescription	1. Provide feedback on lab results, blood pressure control, changes in weight to patient and/or caregiver as is appropriate. 2. Provide feedback on appropriateness of nutrition support and food choices and portions to patient and/or caregiver as is appropriate. 3. Recommend changes in nutrient intake amounts or methods of feeding that may improve outcomes. 4. Adjust MNT, as is appropriate.
Self-Management Skills	1. Review and reinforce self-management skills from prior session. 2. Provide and review educational materials as is appropriate. 3. If medication change, discuss potential food/drug interaction. 4. Discuss transition to enteral/oral feeding, if appropriate. 5. Assess comprehension of education provided and projected compliance.
Functional Ability	1. Refer to OT, PT, speech therapy as appropriate.
Behavioral Goals	1. Reset short-term behavioral goals that are specific and achievable. 2. Review and reinforce long-term goals. 3. Establish follow-up plan.
Communication	1. Document current nutritional status, plan of care, and goals of MNT. 2. Report recommendations/concerns to appropriate health care team member (e.g., MD, RN, pharmacist, social worker). 3. Provide information regarding nutrition prescription and dietary guidelines to extended-care facility, home health care agencies, if appropriate.

Monthly Nutrition Assessment

Session: *Nutritional Update*   Length: *30–45 minutes*   Time: *Monthly, or as indicated*

Factor	Assessments
Clinical Data	1. Review changes in medical status and recent/planned therapies (e.g., medications, dialysis, surgery). 2. Review any new or updated laboratory data (see Appendix F). 3. Assess changes in dry weight and interdialytic weight changes, if appropriate. 4. Assess muscle and fat stores, presence of edema. 5. Assess for physical signs of nutrient deficiencies/excesses or increased needs (e.g., decubiti, poor wound healing, thinning hair, pale conjunctiva, cheilosis). 6. Review dialysis adequacy and PET results, if available. 7. Determine nitrogen balance using urea kinetics, if appropriate (see Appendix D). 8. Assess blood pressure control. 9. Assess effectiveness of previous nutrition intervention.
Dietary Evaluation	1. Assess tolerance of nutrition support. 2. Determine current GI or feeding issues or concerns. 3. Assess changes in ability to digest, absorb, and tolerate oral intake. 4. Assess bowel function (e.g., diarrhea, constipation, ostomy output). 5. Determine use of vitamin/mineral, herbal, or other nutrition supplements. 6. For PD, determine glucose absorption and calories from dialysate (see Appendix C). 7. Determine fluid intake/output and hydration status. 8. Assess intake of calories, protein, sodium, potassium, phosphorus, calcium, and other nutrients as indicated. 9. Assess diet order, tube-feeding order, parenteral nutrition order, and/or IDPN/IPN order for appropriateness.
Functional Ability	1. Determine level of functional ability and recent changes. 2. Assess ability to feed self and needs for assistance. 3. Assess changes in activity level.
Psychosocial and Economic Issues	1. Assess changes in living situation, cooking facilities, finances, education, employment, literacy, and other factors that may affect availability of food or ability to provide safe nutritional support at home, if appropriate. 2. Assess availability of support systems. 3. Determine whether other relevant psychosocial or economic issues exist that impact provision of nutritional support.
Behavioral Outcomes	1. Assess understanding of prior nutritional support education and recommended prescription. 2. Assess understanding of food/drug interactions. 3. Assess understanding of transition to enteral/oral feeding, if appropriate. 4. Determine further improvements that can be made in the quality of the nutritional support care that is being provided.
Behavioral Goals	1. Assess achievement of prior behavioral goals. 2. Determine willingness and ability to make further changes.

Monthly Nutrition Intervention

Session: *Nutritional Update*   Length: *45–60 minutes*   Time: *Monthly, or as indicated*

Factor	Interventions
Management Goals	1. Reassess and adjust management goals of patient and health care team.
Nutrition Prescription	1. Provide feedback on lab results, blood pressure control, changes in weight to patient and/or caregiver. 2. Provide feedback on appropriateness of nutrition support and food choices and portions to patient and/or caregiver. 3. Assess need for continued nutrition support or change in nutritional support method. 4. Recommend changes in nutrient intake amounts or methods of feeding that may improve outcomes. 5. Adjust MNT as is appropriate.
Self-Management Skills	1. Review and reinforce self-management skills. 2. Provide and review educational materials as is appropriate. 3. If medication change, discuss potential food/drug interaction. 4. Discuss transition to enteral/oral feeding, if appropriate. 5. Assess comprehension of education provided and projected compliance.
Functional Ability	1. Provide necessary referrals for assistance with self-feeding and other activities of daily living (e.g., OT, PT, speech therapy).
Behavioral Goals	1. Reset short-term behavioral goals that are specific and achievable. 2. Review and reinforce long-term goals. 3. Establish follow-up plan.
Communication	1. Document current nutritional status, plan of care, and goals of MNT. 2. Report recommendations/concerns to appropriate health care team member (e.g., MD, RN, pharmacist, social worker). 3. Provide information regarding nutrition prescription and dietary guidelines to extended-care facility, home health care agencies, if appropriate.

Bibliography

American Dietetic Association. *Handbook of Clinical Dietetics.* 2nd ed. New Haven, Conn: Yale University Press; 1992.

American Society for Parenteral and Enteral Nutrition. Standards for home nutrition support. *Nutr Clin Pract.* 1992;7:65–69.

Bailey JL, Mitch WE. The implications of metabolic acidosis in intensive care unit patients. *Nephrol Dial Transplant.* 1998;13:837–839.

Bargman JM. The rationale and ultimate limitations of urea kinetic modelling in the estimation of nutritional status. *Peritoneal Dial Int.* 1996;16:347–351.

Campbell SM, Hall J, Krupp K. *Enteral Nutrition Handbook.* Columbus, Ohio: Ross Products Division, Abbott Laboratories; 1995.

Cato Y. Intradialytic parenteral nutrition therapy for the malnourished hemodialysis patient. *J Intravenous Nurs.* 1997;20(3):130–135.

Chertow GM, Bullard A, Lazarus JM. Nutrition and the dialysis prescription. *Am J Nephrol.* 1996;16:79–89.

Chertow GM, Ling J, Lew NL, Lazarus JM, Lowrie EG. The Association of intradialytic parenteral nutrition administration with survival in hemodialysis patients. *Am J Kidney Dis.* 1994;24(6):912–920.

The Chicago Dietetic Association and The South Suburban Dietetic Association. *Manual of Clinical Dietetics.* 5th ed. Chicago, Ill: The American Dietetic Association; 1996.

Compher C, Mullen JL, Barker CF. Nutritional support in renal failure. *Surg Clin N Am.* 1991; 71(3):597–608.

Cotton AB. Enteral nutrition in the dialysis patient. *Diet Curr.* 1995;22(1):1–4.

Daugirdas JT, Ing TS. *Handbook of Dialysis.* 2nd ed. Boston, Mass: Little, Brown; 1994.

Dureke TB, Barany P, Cazzola M, Eschbach W, Grutzmacher P, Kaltwasser JP, Macdougall IC, Pippard MJ, Shaldon S, van Wyck D. Management of iron deficiency in renal anemia: Guidelines for the optimal therapeutic approach in erythropoietin-treated patients. *Clin Nephrol.* 1997; 48(1):1–8.

Emery E, Liftman C. Enteral feedings for renal patients: A primer. *Renal Nutr Forum.* 1997; 16(2):1–3, 8.

Evans MA, Liffrig TK, Nelson JK, Compher C. Home nutrition support patient education materials. *Nutr Clin Pract.* 1993;8:43–47.

Fishbane S, Maesaka JK. Iron management in end-stage renal disease. *Am J Kidney Dis.* 1997; 29(3):319–333.

Fresenius Medical Care/NMC Homecare. *Comprehensive Renal Nutrition Support Program: IDPN/IPN Clinical Manual.* Lexington, Mass: Fresenius Medical Care/NMC Homecare; 1998.

Goldstein DJ, Strom JA. Intradialytic parenteral nutrition: Evolution and current concepts. *J Renal Nutr.* 1991;1(1):9–22.

Gottschlich MM, Matarese LE, Shronts EP, eds. *Nutrition Support Dietetics Core Curriculum.* 2nd ed. Silver Spring, Md: American Society of Parenteral Enteral Nutrition; 1993.

Grant A, DeHoog S. *Nutritional Assessment and Support.* 4th ed. Seattle, Wash: Anne Grant/Susan DeHoog; 1991.

Hirschberg RR, Kopple JD. Energy requirements in patients with renal failure. *Contrib Nephrol.* 1990;81:124–135.

Klein CJ, Stanek GS, Wiles CE. Overfeeding macronutrients to critically ill adults: Metabolic complications. *J Am Diet Assoc.* 1998;98(7):795–806.

Knochel JP. Complications of total parenteral nutrition. *Kidney Int.* 1985;27:489–496.

Kopple JD, Massry SG, eds. *Nutritional Management of Renal Disease.* Baltimore, Md: Williams & Wilkins; 1997.

Matarese LE, Gottschlich MM. *Contemporary Nutrition Support Practice: A Clinical Guide.* Philadelphia, Pa: WB Saunders Company; 1998.

McCann L, ed. *Pocket Guide to Nutritional Assessment of the Adult Renal Patient.* 2nd ed. New York, NY: National Kidney Foundation; 1998.

McCann L. *Subjective Global Assessment.* Redwood City, Calif: Satellite Dialysis Centers, Inc; 1997.

McCann L. Subjective global assessment as it pertains to the nutritional status of dialysis patients. *Dial & Transplant.* 1996;25(4):190–199, 202, 225.

McCann L, Yates L, Ezaki-Yamaguchi J, Akiyama P. Forms to monitor and assess nutritional status of renal patients. *J Renal Nutr.* 1995;5(3):151–155.

Mitch WE. Influence of metabolic acidosis on nutrition. *Am J Kidney Dis.* 1997;29(5):xivi–xiviii.

Movilli E, Bossini N, Viola BF, Camerini C, Cancarini GC, Feller P, Strada A, Maiorca R. Evidence for an independent role of metabolic acidosis on nutritional status in haemodialysis patients. *Nephrol Dial Transplant.* 1998;13:674–678.

Movilli E, Zani R, Carli O, Sangalli L, Pola A, Camerini C, Cancarini GC, Scolari F, Feller P, Maiorca R. Correction of metabolic acidosis increases serum albumin concentrations and decreases kinetically evaluated protein intake in haemodialysis patients: A prospective study. *Nephrol Dial Transplant.* 1998;13:1719–1722.

Nissenson AR. Achieving target hematocrit in dialysis patients: New concepts in iron management. *Am J Kidney Dis.* 1997;30(6):907–911.

Nutritional Support Reference Manual. Seattle, Wash: Harborview Medical Center; 1993.

Schneeweiss R, Graninger W, Stockenhuber F, Druml W, Ferenci P, Eichinger S, Grimm G, Laggner AN, Lenz K. Energy metabolism in acute and chronic renal failure. *Am J Clin Nutr.* 1990;52:596–601.

Stover J (ed). *A Clinical Guide to Nutrition Care in End-Stage Renal Disease.* 2nd ed. Chicago, Ill: American Dietetic Association; 1994.

Sunder-Plassmann G, Horl WH. Erythropoietin and iron. *Clin Nephrol.* 1997;47(3):141–157.

Varella L, Utermohlen V. Nutritional support for the patient with renal failure. *Crit Care Nurs Clin N Amer.* 1993;5(1):79–96.

Winkler M, Lysen LK (eds). *Suggested Guidelines for Nutrition and Metabolic Management of Adult Patients Receiving Nutrition Support.* 2nd ed. Chicago, Ill: The American Dietetic Association; 1993.

Wolfson M, Foulks CJ. Intradialytic parenteral nutrition: A useful therapy? *Nutr Clin Pract.* 1996;11:5–11.

Guideline 4
Nutrition Care of Adult Hospitalized Dialysis Patients

Synopsis/Summary

Diagnosis: End-Stage Renal Disease (Adult 18+ years)

Treatment Mode: Hemodialysis or Peritoneal Dialysis

Setting: Inpatient hospital

Exceptions for Chart Audit: Patients who are younger than 18 years of age; patients who are discharged within 72 hours; patients who transfer to another hospital, or receive transplants; patients for whom intervention is not appropriate; patients who are admitted for graft revision and whose course is uncomplicated. For subjective data, patients who are unwilling or unable to communicate and have no caregivers who wish to do so.

Encounter	Length of Contact	Intervals Between Encounters
Initial	60–90 minutes	Within 72 hours of nutrition referral
Follow-up	30–45 minutes	Daily if high risk; weekly or as indicated if not high risk
Discharge Planning	10–15 minutes	Completed prior to discharge

End-Stage Renal Disease, Hospitalized Dialysis Flowchart

Encounter   **Data/Stage**

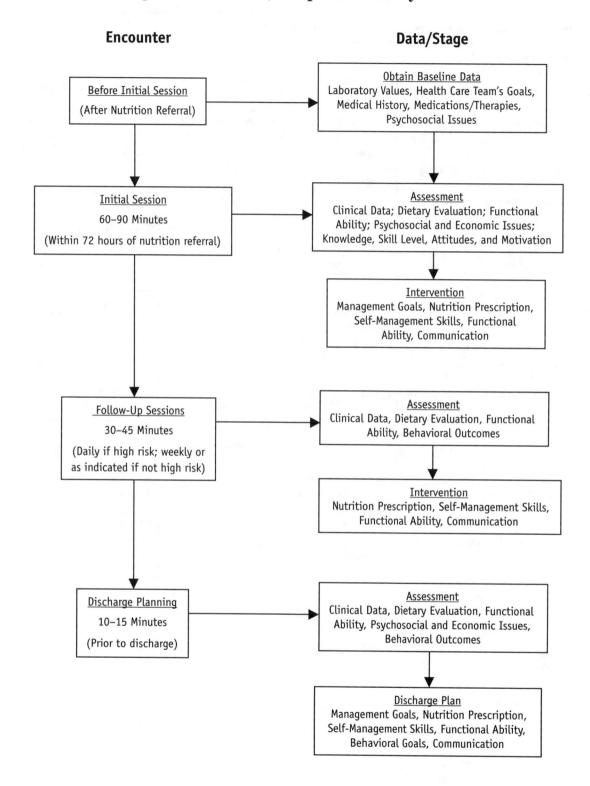

Expected Outcomes of Medical Nutrition Therapy

Outcome Assessment Factors	Expected Outcome of Therapy	Ideal/Goal Value
Clinical Outcomes • Biochemical Parameters —Albumin/prealbumin —Potassium —Phosphorus —Calcium —Serum glucose (casual)	 —Albumin/prealbumin level stabilized or moving toward goal range —Potassium maintained within goal range —Phosphorus and calcium levels progressing toward goal ranges —Blood sugar levels maintained within goal range	 —Albumin $\geq$ 4.0 g/dL, prealbumin $\geq$ 30 mg/dL —Potassium 3.5–5.5 mEq/L —Phosphorus 4.0–6.0 mg/dL —Calcium 8.5–10.5 mg/dL —Serum glucose 80–200 mg/dL
• Hematological Parameters —Hematocrit/hemoglobin —Ferritin —Transferrin saturation	 —Adequate erythropoiesis maintained —Adequate iron stores maintained for erythropoiesis	 —Hematocrit 33–36% hemoglobin 11.0–12.0 g/dL —Ferritin 100–800 ng/mL —Transferrin saturation 20–50%
• Anthropometrics —Dry weight —Interdialytic fluid gains (hemodialysis)	 —Lean body mass preserved —Fluid gains achieved/maintained at goal	 —Within reasonable body weight (BMI 20–25) —Fluid gains 2–5% body weight
• Clinical Signs and Symptoms	—Adequate body mass maintained —Level of functional ability maintained —Good appetite maintained	—Adequate muscle/fat stores —Optimum functional ability —Minimum GI symptoms —Food intake > 80% recommended intake
Patient/Caregiver Behavioral Outcomes • Food selection/meal planning • Potential food/drug interactions	(Prior to discharge) —Verbalizes understanding of diet and demonstrates understanding through correct menu selection, if appropriate —Verbalizes potential food/drug interactions	**MNT Goals** 1. Makes appropriate food choices and takes medications as prescribed 2. Maintains lab values within acceptable limits

Minimum Baseline Data Needed for Medical Nutrition Therapy

Factor	Data Needed
Laboratory Values with Dates and Time of Draw (e.g., pre/post dialysis)	1. BUN, creatinine 2. Albumin/prealbumin 3. Sodium, potassium 4. Phosphorus, calcium, magnesium 5. Serum glucose 6. Hematocrit/hemoglobin 7. Dialysis adequacy and PET results, if available 8. Urea nitrogen appearance (UNA), if available 9. Others as appropriate (e.g., glycosylated hemoglobin, lipid profile, serum bicarbonate, ferritin)
Health Care Team's Goals for Patient	1. Patient prognosis 2. Expected outcome of nutrition therapy 3. Aggressive versus conservative measures
Medical History	1. Reason for hospitalization 2. Disease/condition causing renal failure 3. History of renal disease and treatment 4. Concurrent medical conditions (e.g., diabetes, cancer, HIV, cardiovascular disease, GI problems, hypertension, hyperlipidemia) 5. Any other medical or physical conditions with potential nutritional implications (e.g., surgery, infection, CVA, chemotherapy, blindness, neuropathies)
Medications/Therapies	1. Type of dialysis therapy and prescription 2. Diet order, tube-feeding order, or parenteral nutrition order 3. IV administration (e.g., Calcijex, Imferon, Infed, EPO) 4. Regulation of bowel function 5. Any other therapies/treatments which may affect nutritional intake or status 6. Antihypertensives, diuretics 7. Phosphate binders 8. Anticoagulants 9. Vitamin/mineral supplements 10. Any other medications with food/drug interactions or nutritional impact (e.g., diabetes medications, GI medications, steroids, antibiotics)
Psychosocial Issues (as appropriate)	1. Learning disabilities 2. Vision, hearing abilities 3. Cultural or language barriers 4. Mental status

Initial Nutrition Assessment

Session: *Initial*   Length: *60–90 minutes*   Time: *Within 72 hours of nutrition referral*

Factor	Assessments
Clinical Data	1. Review minimum baseline data. 2. Obtain current height, weight at admission, dry weight, and BMI. 3. Obtain weight history, recent weight changes, and weight goals. 4. Determine IBW and/or UBW adjusted for amputation or obesity, and percentage IBW and/or percentage UBW (see Appendix B). 5. Assess muscle and fat stores, presence of edema. 6. Assess for physical signs of nutrient deficiencies/excesses or increased needs (e.g., decubiti, poor wound healing, thinning hair, pale conjunctiva, cheilosis).
Dietary Evaluation	1. Determine previous dietary instruction and practices. 2. Determine usual food intake and pattern of intake prior to admission. 3. Assess appetite, GI issues, tolerance of oral intake, and food allergies/intolerances. 4. Assess feeding issues (e.g., chewing, swallowing). 5. Determine use of vitamin/mineral, herbal, or other nutrition supplements. 6. Determine alcohol/drug/tobacco use and history. 7. For PD, determine glucose absorption and calories from dialysate (see Appendix C). 8. Assess intake of calories, protein, sodium, potassium, phosphorus, calcium, fluids, and other nutrients as indicated. 9. Determine need for enteral or parenteral nutrition. 10. Assess diet order, tube-feeding order, parenteral nutrition order, and/or IDPN/IPN order for appropriateness.
Functional Ability	1. Determine level of functional ability and recent changes. 2. Assess ability to feed self and needs for assistance.
Psychosocial and Economic Issues	1. Assess educational background, literacy level, as is appropriate. 2. Assess ethnic or religious belief considerations. 3. Assess availability of support systems. 4. Determine whether other relevant psychosocial or economic issues exist.
Knowledge, Skill Level, Attitudes, and Motivation	1. Assess basic knowledge level of dietary guidelines for patient's mode of treatment. 2. Assess basic knowledge level of impact of renal disease on nutrition.

Initial Nutrition Intervention

Session: *Initial*   Length: *60–90 minutes*   Time: *Within 72 hours of nutrition referral*

Factor	Interventions
Management Goals	1. Identify management goals of health care team. 2. Identify patient goals and expectations.
Nutrition Prescription	1. Calories—individualized; use basal energy expenditure × stress factor; or use 30–35 kcal/kg IBW or adjusted weight (hemodialysis); 25–35 kcal/kg IBW or adjusted weight (peritoneal dialysis-includes calories from dialysate glucose absorption) 2. Protein = 1.1–1.4 g/kg IBW or adjusted weight (hemodialysis); 1.2–1.5 g/kg IBW or adjusted weight (peritoneal dialysis); may be higher depending on stress or metabolic needs 3. Sodium—individualized, approximately 2–3 g/day (hemodialysis); 2–4 g/day (peritoneal dialysis) 4. Potassium—individualized, approximately 40 mg/kg IBW or adjusted weight (hemodialysis); restricted only by lab values (peritoneal dialysis) 5. Phosphorus—individualized, approximately. $\leq$ 17 mg/kg IBW or adjusted weight; may require phosphate binder therapy 6. Calcium—individualized per calcium, phosphorus, and PTH lab values and use of vitamin D; approximately 1000–1500 mg/day 7. Fluids—500–750 mL + urine output per day (or 1000 mL/day if anuric) (hemodialysis); to maintain fluid balance (peritoneal dialysis) 8. Vitamin/mineral supplementation—as appropriate 9. Implement meal/nutrition therapy plan per prescription
Self-Management Skills	1. Discuss nutrition therapy recommendations with patient and/or caregiver. 2. Discuss basic dietary guidelines for ESRD as indicated. 3. Discuss role and effect of diet and medications on renal disease and dialysis treatment, if appropriate. 4. Assess comprehension of education provided and projected compliance.
Functional Ability	1. Provide necessary referrals for assistance with self-feeding and other activities of daily living (e.g., OT, PT, speech therapy).
Communication	1. Document current nutritional status, plan of care, and goals of MNT. 2. Report recommendations/concerns to appropriate health care team member (e.g., MD, RN, pharmacist, social worker).

Follow-up Nutrition Assessment

Session: *Follow-up*   Length: *30–45 minutes*   Time: *Daily if high risk; Weekly or as indicated if not high risk*

Factor	Assessments
Clinical Data	1. Review changes in medical status and recent/planned therapies (e.g., medications, dialysis, surgery). 2. Review any new or updated laboratory data. 3. Assess changes in dry weight, interdialytic weight changes if appropriate, and presence of edema. 4. Assess for physical signs of nutrient deficiencies/excesses or increased needs (e.g., decubiti, poor wound healing, thinning hair, pale conjunctiva, cheilosis). 5. Assess effectiveness of previous nutrition intervention.
Dietary Evaluation	1. Determine current GI or feeding issues or concerns, tolerance of oral intake. 2. Assess changes in patient's food intake and/or appetite. 3. Determine fluid intake/output and hydration status. 4. For CAVH or PD, determine glucose absorption and calories from dialysate (see Appendix C). 5. Assess dietary intake and/or nutritional support for adequacy and appropriateness.
Functional Ability	1. Assess changes in functional ability. 2. Assess changes in activity level, if appropriate.
Behavioral Outcomes	1. Assess understanding of nutrition therapy recommendations. 2. Assess understanding of basic dietary guidelines for ESRD. 3. Assess understanding of role and effect of diet and medications on renal disease and dialysis treatment, if appropriate.

Follow-up Nutrition Intervention

Session: *Follow-up*   Length: *30–45 minutes*   Time: *Daily if high risk; Weekly or as indicated if not high risk*

Factor	Interventions
Nutrition Prescription	1. Recommend changes in nutrient intake amounts or methods of feeding that may improve outcomes. 2. Adjust MNT, as is appropriate.
Self-Management Skills	1. Discuss nutrition therapy changes and recommendations with patient and/or caregiver as indicated. 2. Assess comprehension of education provided and projected compliance.
Functional Ability	1. Refer to OT, PT, speech therapy as is appropriate.
Communication	1. Document current nutritional status, plan of care, and goals of MNT. 2. Report recommendations/concerns to appropriate health care team member (e.g., MD, RN, pharmacist, social worker).

Discharge Nutrition Assessment

Session: *Discharge Planning*   Length: *10–15 minutes*   Time: *Prior to discharge*

Factor	Assessments
Clinical Data	1. Review changes in medical status and recent/planned therapies (e.g., medications, dialysis, surgery). 2. Review any new or updated laboratory data. 3. Assess changes in dry weight and interdialytic weight changes. 4. Assess muscle and fat stores, presence of edema. 5. Assess for physical signs of nutrient deficiencies/excesses or increased needs (e.g., decubiti, poor wound healing, thinning hair, pale conjunctiva, cheilosis).
Dietary Evaluation	1. Determine current GI or feeding issues or concerns, tolerance of oral intake. 2. Assess changes in patient's food intake and/or appetite. 3. Determine fluid intake/output and hydration status. 4. For CAVH or PD, determine glucose absorption and calories from dialysate (see Appendix C). 5. Assess dietary intake and/or nutritional support intake for adequacy and appropriateness.
Functional Ability	1. Determine level of functional ability and recent changes. 2. Assess ability to feed self and needs for assistance.
Psychosocial and Economic Issues	1. Assess living situation, cooking facilities, finances, educational background, employment, literacy, and other factors that may affect availability of food. 2. Assess availability of support systems. 3. Determine whether other relevant psychosocial or economic issues exist.
Behavioral Outcomes	1. Assess understanding of nutrition therapy guidelines and recommended food/meal plan. 2. Assess understanding of relevant food/drug interactions. 3. Determine further improvements that can be made in the quality of the diet.

Discharge Plan

Session: *Discharge Planning*   Length: *10–15 minutes*   Time: *Prior to discharge*

Factor	Interventions
Management Goals	1. Reassess and adjust management goals of patient and health care team.
Nutrition Prescription	1. Provide feedback on lab results, changes in weight to patient and/or caregiver as appropriate. 2. Provide feedback on food/meal plan, food choices, and portions to patient and/or caregiver as is appropriate. 3. Recommend changes in nutrient intake or habits that may improve outcomes. 4. Adjust MNT, as is appropriate.
Self-Management Skills	1. Review and reinforce self-management skills. 2. Provide and review nutrition educational materials as is appropriate. 3. If medication change, discuss potential food/drug interaction. 4. Discuss use and effect of phosphate binders, if appropriate. 5. Discuss dry weight and fluid restrictions if appropriate. 6. Assess comprehension of education provided and projected compliance.
Functional Ability	1. Provide necessary referrals for assistance with self-feeding and other activities of daily living (e.g., OT, PT, speech therapy).
Behavioral Goals	1. Set behavioral goals that are specific and achievable. 2. Determine willingness and ability to meet behavioral goals.
Communication	1. Provide information regarding nutrition prescription and dietary guidelines to dialysis facility, extended-care facility, home health care agencies, and/or primary care physician. 2. Provide patient with referral for follow-up nutrition services, as is appropriate.

Bibliography

American Diabetes Association Position Statement: Hospital Admission Guidelines for Diabetes Mellitus. *Diabetes Care.* 1997;20(Suppl 1):S52.

American Diabetes Association Position Statement: Translation of the Diabetes Nutrition Recommendations for Health Care Institutions. *Diabetes Care.* 1997;20(Suppl 1):S37–S39.

Bailey JL, Mitch WE. The implications of metabolic acidosis in intensive care unit patients. *Nephrol Dial Transplant.* 1998;13:837–839.

Bargman JM. The rationale and ultimate limitations of urea kinetic modelling in the estimation of nutritional status. *Peritoneal Dial Int.* 1996;16:347–351.

Bourke E, Delaney V. Assessment of hypocalcemia and hypercalcemia. *Clin in Lab Med.* 1993; 13(1):157–181.

Chicago Dietetic Association, South Suburban Dietetic Association, Dietitians of Canada. *Manual of Clinical Dietetics.* 6th ed. Chicago, Ill: American Dietetic Association; 2000.

Daugirdas JT, Ing TS. *Handbook of Dialysis.* 2nd ed. Boston, Mass: Little, Brown; 1994.

Gottschlich MM, Matarese LE, Shronts EP (eds). *Nutrition Support Dietetics Core Curriculum.* 2nd ed. Silver Spring, Md: American Society of Parenteral Enteral Nutrition; 1993.

Grant A, DeHoog S. *Nutritional Assessment and Support.* 4th ed. Seattle, Wash: Anne Grant/Susan DeHoog; 1991.

Hirschberg RR, Kopple JD. Energy requirements in patients with renal failure. *Contrib Nephrol.* 1990;81:124–135.

Klein CJ, Stanek GS, Wiles CE. Overfeeding macronutrients to critically ill adults: Metabolic complications. *J Am Diet Assoc.* 1998;98(7):795–806.

Kopple JD, Massry SG, eds. *Nutritional Management of Renal Disease.* Baltimore, Md: Williams & Wilkins; 1997.

Manning EMC, Shenkin A. Nutritional assessment in the critically ill. *Crit Care Clin.* 1995;11(3): 603–635.

McCann L, ed. *Pocket Guide to Nutritional Assessment of the Adult Renal Patient.* 2nd ed. New York, NY: National Kidney Foundation; 1998.

Movilli E, Bossini N, Viola BF, Camerini C, Cancarini GC, Feller P, Strada A, Maiorca R. Evidence for an independent role of metabolic acidosis on nutritional status in haemodialysis patients. *Nephrol Dial Transplant.* 1998;13:674–678.

Movilli E, Zani R, Carli O, Sangalli L, Pola A, Camerini C, Cancarini GC, Scolari F, Feller P, Maiorca R. Correction of metabolic acidosis increases serum albumin concentrations and decreases kinetically evaluated protein intake in haemodialysis patients: A prospective study. *Nephrol Dial Transplant.* 1998;13:1719–1722.

Nutritional Support Reference Manual. Seattle, Wash: Harborview Medical Center; 1993.

Schneeweiss R, Graninger W, Stockenhuber F, Druml W, Ferenci P, Eichinger S, Grimm G, Laggner AN, Lenz K. Energy metabolism in acute and chronic renal failure. *Am J Clin Nutr.* 1990;52:596–601.

Stover J, ed. *A Clinical Guide to Nutrition Care in End-Stage Renal Disease.* 2nd ed. Chicago, Ill:American Dietetic Association; 1994.

Varella L, Utermohlen V. Nutritional support for the patient with renal failure. *Crit Care Nurs Clin N Am.* 1993;5(1):79–96.

Guideline 5
Nutrition Care of Adult Acute Renal Failure Patients

Synopsis/Summary

Diagnosis: Acute Renal Failure (Adult 18+ years)

Setting: In-patient hospital

Exceptions for Chart Audit: Patients who are younger than 18 years of age; patients who are discharged within 72 hours; patients who transfer to another hospital, or receive transplants; patients for whom nutrition intervention is not appropriate (e.g., hospice, palliative care, poor prognosis). For subjective data, patients who are unwilling or unable to communicate and have no caregivers who wish to do so.

Encounter	Length of Contact	Intervals Between Encounters
Initial	60–90 minutes	Within 72 hours of nutrition referral
Follow-up	30–45 minutes	Daily, or as indicated
Discharge Planning	10–15 minutes	Completed prior to discharge

Adult Acute Renal Failure Flowchart

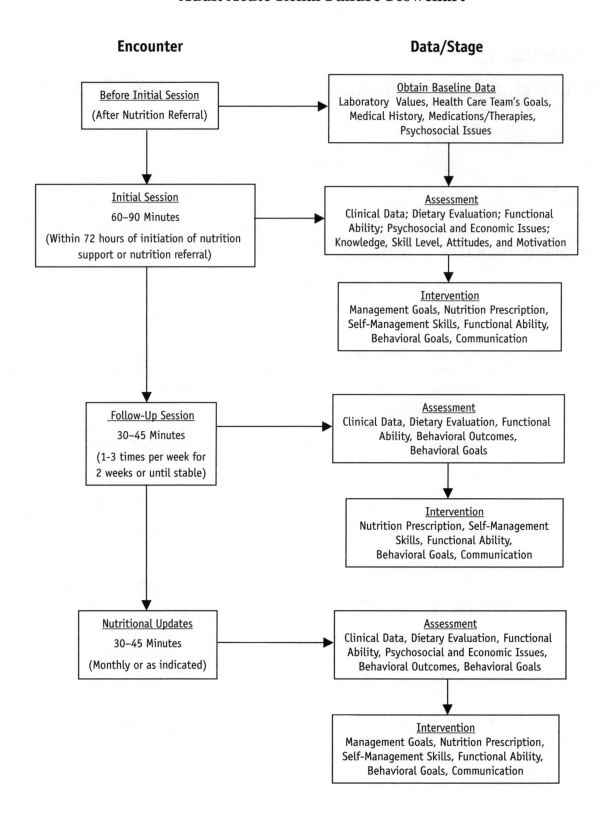

Encounter

Data/Stage

Before Initial Session
(After Nutrition Referral)

Obtain Baseline Data
Laboratory Values, Health Care Team's Goals, Medical History, Medications/Therapies, Psychosocial Issues

Initial Session
60–90 Minutes
(Within 72 hours of initiation of nutrition support or nutrition referral)

Assessment
Clinical Data; Dietary Evaluation; Functional Ability; Psychosocial and Economic Issues; Knowledge, Skill Level, Attitudes, and Motivation

Intervention
Management Goals, Nutrition Prescription, Self-Management Skills, Functional Ability, Behavioral Goals, Communication

Follow-Up Session
30–45 Minutes
(1-3 times per week for 2 weeks or until stable)

Assessment
Clinical Data, Dietary Evaluation, Functional Ability, Behavioral Outcomes, Behavioral Goals

Intervention
Nutrition Prescription, Self-Management Skills, Functional Ability, Behavioral Goals, Communication

Nutritional Updates
30–45 Minutes
(Monthly or as indicated)

Assessment
Clinical Data, Dietary Evaluation, Functional Ability, Psychosocial and Economic Issues, Behavioral Outcomes, Behavioral Goals

Intervention
Management Goals, Nutrition Prescription, Self-Management Skills, Functional Ability, Behavioral Goals, Communication

Expected Outcomes of Medical Nutrition Therapy

Outcome Assessment Factors	Expected Outcome of Therapy	Ideal/Goal Value

Clinical Outcomes
• Biochemical Parameters
  —Albumin/prealbumin
 	
  —Sodium
  —Potassium
  —Phosphorus
  —Calcium
  —Magnesium
 	
  —Serum glucose (casual)
 	
  —Triglycerides (if on TPN)
 	
  —Chloride
  —CO_2
	—Albumin/prealbumin levels stabilized or moving toward goal range
	—Sodium and potassium levels maintained within goal ranges
	—Phosphorus, calcium, magnesium levels maintained within goal ranges
	
	—Blood sugar levels maintained within goal range
	—Triglycerides maintained within goal range
	
	—Chloride and CO_2 levels within goal ranges
		—Albumin 3.5–5.0 g/dL, prealbumin 19–43 mg/dL
		—Sodium 135–145 mEq/L
		—Potassium 3.5–5.5 mEq/L
		—Phosphorus 2.5–6.0 mg/dL
		—Calcium 8.5–10.5 mg/dL
		—Magnesium 1.5–2.0 mEq/L
		—Serum glucose 80–200 mg/dL (enteral), 150–250 mg/dL (parenteral)
		—Triglycerides < 250 mg/dL 4 hrs after lipids stopped, < 400 mg/dL during continuous infusion
		—Chloride 100–106 mEq/L
		—CO_2 24–30 mEq/L

• Hematological Parameters
  —Hematocrit/hemoglobin
 	
  —Ferritin
  —Transferrin saturation
	—Adequate erythropoiesis maintained
	
	—Adequate iron stores maintained for erythropoiesis
		—Hematocrit 36–45% (F), 38–50% (M) hemoglobin 12–16 g/dL (F), 14–18 g/dL (M)
		—Ferritin 100–800 ng/mL
		—Transferrin saturation 20–50%

• Anthropometrics —Weight • Clinical Signs and Symptoms	—Lean body mass preserved —Adequate body mass maintained —Level of functional ability maintained —Good appetite maintained	—Within reasonable body weight (BMI 20–25) —Adequate muscle/fat stores —Optimum functional ability —Minimum GI symptoms —Food intake > 80% recommended intake
Patient/Caregiver Behavioral Outcomes • Food selection/meal planning • Potential food/drug interactions	(Prior to discharge) —Verbalizes understanding of diet and demonstrates understanding through correct menu selection, if appropriate —Verbalizes potential food/drug interactions	**MNT Goals** 1. Makes appropriate food choices and takes medications as prescribed 2. Maintains lab values within acceptable limits

Minimum Baseline Data Needed for Medical Nutrition Therapy

Factor	Data Needed
Laboratory Values with Dates	1. BUN, creatinine 2. Albumin/prealbumin 3. Sodium, potassium 4. Phosphorus, calcium, magnesium 5. Serum glucose 6. Serum chloride, CO_2 7. Hematocrit/hemoglobin 8. Urinalysis results (e.g., volume, urea, protein, sodium) 9. Others as appropriate (e.g., triglycerides, ferritin)
Health Care Team's Goals for Patient	1. Patient prognosis, degree of renal failure, and expected course of renal failure 2. Expected outcome of nutrition therapy 3. Aggressive versus conservative measures
Medical History	1. Reason for hospitalization 2. Disease/condition leading to acute renal failure 3. History of renal disease and treatment 4. Concurrent medical conditions (e.g., diabetes, cancer, HIV, cardiovascular disease, GI problems, hypertension, hyperlipidemia) 5. Any other medical or physical conditions with potential nutritional implications (e.g., surgery, infection, CVA, chemotherapy)
Medications/Therapies	1. Type of dialysis therapy and prescription, if appropriate 2. Diet order, tube-feeding order, or parenteral nutrition order 3. IV administration 4. Regulation of bowel function 5. Any other therapies/treatments that may affect nutritional intake or status (e.g., ventilation) 6. Antihypertensives, diuretics 7. Anticoagulants 8. Vitamin/mineral supplements 9. Any other medications with food/drug interactions or nutritional impact (e.g., diabetes medications, GI medications, steroids, phosphate binders, antibiotics)
Psychosocial Issues (as appropriate)	1. Learning disabilities 2. Vision, hearing abilities 3. Cultural or language barriers 4. Mental status

Initial Nutrition Assessment

Session: *Initial*   Length: *60–90 minutes*   Time: *Within 72 hours of nutrition referral*

Factor	Assessments
Clinical Data	1. Review minimum baseline data. 2. Obtain current height, weight at admission, estimated dry weight, and BMI. 3. Obtain weight history, recent weight changes, and weight goals. 4. Determine IBW and/or UBW adjusted for amputation or obesity, and percentage IBW and/or percentage UBW (see Appendix B). 5. Assess muscle and fat stores, presence of edema. 6. Assess for physical signs of nutrient deficiencies/excesses or increased needs (e.g., decubiti, poor wound healing, thinning hair, pale conjunctiva, cheilosis). 7. Determine nitrogen balance using urea kinetics, if appropriate (see Appendix D).
Dietary Evaluation	1. Determine usual food intake and pattern of intake prior to admission. 2. Assess appetite, GI issues, tolerance of oral intake, and food allergies/intolerances. 3. Assess feeding issues (e.g., chewing, swallowing). 4. Determine use of vitamin/mineral, herbal, or other nutrition supplements. 5. Determine alcohol/drug/tobacco use and history. 6. For CAVH and PD, determine glucose absorption and calories from dialysate (see Appendix C). 7. Determine hydration status and assess fluid intake/output. 8. Assess intake of calories, protein, sodium, potassium, phosphorus, calcium, and other nutrients as indicated. 9. Determine need for enteral or parenteral nutrition. 10. Assess diet order, tube-feeding order, and/or parenteral nutrition order for appropriateness.
Functional Ability	1. Determine level of functional ability and recent changes. 2. Assess ability to feed self and needs for assistance.
Psychosocial and Economic Issues	1. Assess ethnic or religious belief considerations. 2. Assess availability of support systems . 3. Determine whether other relevant psychosocial or economic issues exist.

Initial Nutrition Intervention

Session: *Initial*   Length: *60–90 minutes*   Time: *Within 72 hours of nutrition referral*

Factor	Interventions
Management Goals	1. Identify management goals of health care team. 2. Identify patient goals and expectations.
Nutrition Prescription	1. Calories—individualized; determine via indirect calorimetry, if available, or use basal energy expenditure × stress factor, or 30–40 kcal/kg IBW or adjusted weight 2. Protein = 0.5–0.8 g/kg IBW or adjusted weight with no dialysis; 1.0–2.0 g/kg IBW or adjusted weight with dialysis (based on underlying disease state and type of renal replacement therapy) 3. Sodium—*Anuric/oliguric phase*: < 2000 mg/day *Diuretic phase*: replace losses depending on urinary output, edema, dialysis, and serum sodium levels. 4. Potassium—*Anuric/oliguric phase*: individualized per laboratory values *Diuretic phase*: individualized-may need to replace losses depending on urinary volume, serum and urinary potassium levels, frequency of dialysis, and drug therapy. 5. Phosphorus—individualized per laboratory values 6. Calcium—individualized per laboratory values 7. Magnesium—for those receiving nutritional support, individualized per laboratory values 8. Fluids—*Anuric/oliguric phase*: 500 mL + total output (urine, vomitus, and diarrhea) per day *Diuretic phase*: large amounts of fluid may be needed. Assess daily. 9. Vitamin/mineral supplementation—as appropriate 10. Implement nutrition therapy plan per prescription.
Self-Management Skills	1. Discuss nutrition therapy recommendations with patient and/or caregiver. 2. Discuss basic dietary guidelines as indicated and reinforce temporary nature of dietary recommendations as based on medical condition. 3. Discuss role and effect of diet and medications on renal disease and dialysis treatment, if appropriate. 4. Assess comprehension of education provided and projected compliance.
Functional Ability	1. Provide necessary referrals for assistance with self-feeding and other activities of daily living (e.g., OT, PT, speech therapy).
Communication	1. Document current nutritional status, plan of care, and goals of MNT. 2. Report recommendations/concerns to appropriate health care team member (e.g., MD, RN, pharmacist, social worker).

Follow-up Nutrition Assessment

Session: *Follow-up*   Length: *30–45 minutes*   Time: *Daily, or as indicated*

Factor	Assessments
Clinical Data	1. Review changes or expected changes in renal function (e.g., creatinine clearance, GFR, urine output). 2. Review changes in medical status and recent/planned therapies (e.g., medications, dialysis, surgery). 3. Review any new or updated laboratory data. 4. Assess changes in weight and presence of edema. 5. Assess for physical signs of nutrient deficiencies/excesses or increased needs (e.g., decubiti, poor wound healing, thinning hair, pale conjunctiva, cheilosis). 6. Determine nitrogen balance using urea kinetics, if appropriate (see Appendix D). 7. Assess effectiveness of previous nutrition intervention.
Dietary Evaluation	1. Determine current GI or feeding issues or concerns, tolerance of oral intake. 2. Assess changes in patient's food intake and/or appetite. 3. Determine fluid intake/output and hydration status. 4. For CAVH or PD, determine glucose absorption and calories from dialysate (see Appendix C). 5. Assess dietary intake and/or nutritional support for adequacy and appropriateness.
Functional Ability	1. Assess changes in functional ability. 2. Assess changes in activity level.
Behavioral Outcomes	1. Assess understanding of nutrition therapy recommendations. 2. Assess understanding of basic dietary guidelines. 3. Assess understanding of role and effect of diet and medications on renal disease and dialysis treatment.

Follow-up Nutrition Intervention

Session: *Follow-up*   Length: *30–45 minutes*   Time: *Daily, or as indicated*

Factor	Interventions
Nutrition Prescription	1. Recommend changes in nutrient intake amounts or methods of feeding that may improve outcomes. 2. Adjust MNT, as appropriate.
Self-Management Skills	1. Discuss nutrition therapy changes and recommendations with patient and/or caregiver as appropriate. 2. Assess comprehension of education provided and projected compliance.
Functional Ability	1. Refer to OT, PT, speech therapy as appropriate.
Communication	1. Document current nutritional status, plan of care, and goals of MNT. 2. Report recommendations/concerns to appropriate health care team member (e.g., MD, RN, pharmacist, social worker).

Discharge Nutrition Assessment

Session: *Discharge Planning*   Length: *10–15 minutes*   Time: *Prior to discharge*

Factor	Assessments
Clinical Data	1. Review changes or expected changes in renal function (e.g., creatinine clearance, GFR, urine output). 2. Review changes in medical status and recent/planned therapies (e.g., medications, dialysis, surgery). 3. Review any new or updated laboratory data. 5. Assess changes in weight. 6. Assess muscle and fat stores, presence of edema. 7. Assess for physical signs of nutrient deficiencies/excesses or increased needs (e.g., decubiti, poor wound healing, thinning hair, pale conjunctiva, cheilosis).
Dietary Evaluation	1. Determine current GI or feeding issues or concerns, tolerance of oral intake. 2. Assess changes in patient's food intake and/or appetite. 3. Determine fluid intake/output hydration status. 4. For CAVH or PD, determine glucose absorption and calories from dialysate (see Appendix C). 5. Assess dietary intake and/or nutrition support intake for adequacy and appropriateness.
Functional Ability	1. Determine level of functional ability and recent changes. 2. Assess ability to feed self and needs for assistance.
Psychosocial and Economic Issues	1. Assess living situation, cooking facilities, finances, educational background, employment, literacy, and other factors that may affect availability of food. 2. Assess availability of support systems. 3. Determine whether other relevant psychosocial or economic issues exist.
Behavioral Outcomes	1. Assess understanding of nutrition therapy guidelines and recommended food/meal plan. 2. Assess understanding of relevant food/drug interactions. 3. Determine further improvements that can be made in the quality of the diet.

Discharge Plan

Session: *Discharge Planning*   Length: *10–15 minutes*   Time: *Prior to discharge*

Factor	Interventions
Management Goals	1. Reassess and adjust management goals of patient and health care team.
Nutrition Prescription	1. Provide feedback on lab results, changes in weight to patient and/or caregiver as appropriate. 2. Provide feedback on food/meal plan, food choices, and portions to patient and/or caregiver as appropriate. 3. Recommend changes in nutrient intake or habits that may improve outcomes. 4. Adjust MNT, as appropriate.
Self-Management Skills	1. Review and reinforce self-management skills. 2. Provide and review nutrition educational materials as appropriate. 3. If medication change, discuss potential food/drug interaction. 4. Assess comprehension of education provided and projected compliance.
Functional Ability	1. Provide necessary referrals for assistance with self-feeding and other activities of daily living (e.g., OT, PT, speech therapy).
Behavioral Goals	1. Set behavioral goals that are specific and achievable. 2. Determine willingness and ability to meet behavioral goals.
Communication	1. Provide information regarding nutrition prescription and dietary guidelines to dialysis facility, extended-care facility, home health care agencies, and/or primary care physician. 2. Provide patient with referral for follow-up nutrition services, as appropriate.

Bibliography

Alvestrand A. Nutritional aspects in patients with acute renal failure/multiorgan failure. *BloodPurif.* 1996;14:109–114.

Bailey JL, Mitch WE. The implications of metabolic acidosis in intensive care unit patients. *NephrolDialTransplant.* 1998;13:837–839.

Bajapi S. Nutrition in acute renal failure. *RenalNutrForum.* 1998;17(4):1–7.

Bellomo R, Martin H, Parkin G, Love J, Kearley Y, Boyce N. Continuous arteriovenous haemodi-afiltration in the critically ill: Influence on major nutrient balances. *IntensiveCareMed.* 1991;17: 399–402.

Bourke E, Delaney V. Assessment of hypocalcemia and hypercalcemia. *ClinLabMed.* 1993;13(1): 157–181.

Butler BA. Nutritional management of catabolic acute renal failure requiring renal replacement therapy. *ANNAJ.* 1991;18(3):247–259.

Chertow GM, Bullard A, Lazarus JM. Nutrition and the dialysis prescription. *AmJNephrol.* 1996;16:79–89.

Chicago Dietetic Association, South Suburban Dietetic Association, Dietitians of Canada. *Manual of Clinical Dietetics.* 6th ed. Chicago, Ill: American Dietetic Association; 2000.

Chima CS, Meyer L, Heyka R, Bosworth C, Hummel AC, Werynski A, Paganini E, Verdi P. Nitrogen balance in postsurgical patients with acute renal failure on continuous arteriovenous hemofiltration and total parenteral nutrition. *ContribNephrol.* 1991;93:39–41.

Chima CS, Meyer L, Hummell AC, Bosworth C, Heyka R, Paganini EP, Werynski A. Protein catabolic rate in patients with acute renal failure on continuous arteriovenous hemofiltration and total parenteral nutrition. *J AmSocNephrol.* 1993;3:1516–1521.

Compher C, Mullen JL, Barker CF. Nutritional support in renal failure. *SurgClinNAm.* 1991;71(3): 597–608.

Daugirdas JT, Ing TS. *Handbook of Dialysis.* 2nd ed. Boston, Mass: Little, Brown; 1994.

Druml W. Protein metabolism in acute renal failure. *MinerElectrolyteMetab.* 1998;24:47–54.

Druml W. Nutritional considerations in the treatment of acute renal failure in septic patients. *NephrolDialTransplant.* 1994;9(Suppl) 4:219–223.

Goldstein DJ. Nutrition for acute renal failure patients on continuous hemofiltration. *NutrClinPract.* 1988;3:238–241.

Gottschlich MM, Matarese LE, Shronts EP (eds). *Nutrition Support Dietetics Core Curriculum.* 2nd ed. Silver Spring, Md: American Society of Parenteral Enteral Nutrition; 1993.

Hirschberg RR, Kopple JD. Energy requirements in patients with renal failure. *ContribNephrol.* 1990;81:124–135.

Klein CJ, Stanek GS, Wiles CE. Overfeeding macronutrients to critically ill adults: Metabolic complications. *JAmDietAssoc.* 1998;98(7):795–806.

Kopple JD. Nutritional management of acute renal failure. In Kopple JD, Massry SG (eds). *Nutritional Management of Renal Disease.* Baltimore, Md: Williams & Wilkins; 1997.

Macias WL, Alaka KJ, Murphy MH, Miller ME, Clark WR, Mueller BA. Impact of the nutritional regimen on protein catabolism and nitrogen balance in patients with acute renal failure. *JParenteralEnteralNutr.* 1996;20(1):56–62.

Manning EMC, Shenkin A. Nutritional assessment in the critically ill. *CritCareClin.* 1995;11(3): 603–635.

Matarese LE, Gottschlich MM. *Contemporary Nutrition Support Practice: A Clinical Guide.* Philadelphia, Pa: W.B. Saunders Company; 1998.

Molina MF, Riella MC. Nutritional support in the patient with renal failure. *CritCareClin.* 1995;11(3):685–704.

Monaghan R, Watters JM, Clancey SM, Moulton SB, Rabin EZ. Uptake of glucose during continuous arteriovenous hemofiltration. *CritCareMed.* 1993;21(8):1159–1163.

Monson P, Mehta RL. Nutrition in acute renal failure: A reappraisal for the 1990's. *JRenalNutr.* 1994;4(2):58–77.

Nutritional Support Reference Manual. Seattle, Wash: Harborview Medical Center; 1993.

Oldrizzi L, Rugiu C, Maschio G. Nutrition and the kidney: How to manage patients with renal failure. *NutrClinPract.* 1994;9:3–10.

Paganini EP, Derhgawen S. Continuous renal replacement therapy: basic review and clinical considerations. In Kopple JD, Massry SG (eds). *Nutritional Management of Renal Disease.* Baltimore, Md: Williams & Wilkins; 1997.

Rodriguez D, Lewis SL. Nutritional management of patients with acute renal failure. *ANNAJ.* 1997;24(2):232–241.

Schneeweiss R, Graninger W, Stockenhuber F, Druml W, Ferenci P, Eichinger S, Grimm G, Laggner AN, Lenz K. Energy metabolism in acute and chronic renal failure. *AmJClinNutr.* 1990;52:596–601.

Seidner DL, Matarese LE, Steiger E. Nutritional care of the critically ill patient with renal failure. *SeminNephrol.* 1994;14(1):53–63.

Sponsel H, Conger JD. Is parenteral nutrition therapy of value in acute renal failure patients? *AmJKidney Dis.* 1995;25(1):96–102.

Stover J, ed. *A Clinical Guide to Nutrition Care in End-Stage Renal Disease* 2nd ed. Chicago, Ill: The American Dietetic Association; 1994.

Varella L, Utermohlen V. Nutritional support for the patient with renal failure. *CritCareNursClin-NAmer.* 1993;5(1):79–96.

Weiner Feldman RJ. Nutrition in acute renal failure. *JRenalNutr.* 1994;4(2):97–99.

Winkler M, Lysen LK, eds. *Suggested Guidelines for Nutrition and Metabolic Management of Adult Patients Receiving Nutrition Support.* 2nd ed. Chicago, Ill: The American Dietetic Association; 1993.

Guideline 6
Nutrition Care of Adult Transplant Patients

Synopsis/Summary

Diagnosis: Kidney Transplant (Adult 18+ years)

Setting: Transplant Clinic

Exceptions for Chart Audit: Patients who are younger than 18 years of age, patients who die within the first week after transplant, patients who transfer to another facility, patients followed in an outpatient transplant clinic who are re-hospitalized. For subjective data, patients who are unable or unwilling to communicate and have no caregivers who wish to do so.

Encounter	Length of Contact	Intervals Between Encounters
Pretransplant Evaluation	60–90 minutes	Prior to transplantation
Acute Phase Initial*	45–60 minutes	Within 72 hours of transplant
Acute Follow-Up	15–30 minutes	As indicated
Chronic Phase Initial[†]	45–60 minutes	1–2 months post-transplant, as indicated by graft function
Chronic Follow-up	30–45 minutes	6 months following initial and as indicated

*Acute phase:** Immediately posttransplant (up to 4–8 weeks after transplant). Goals are to maintain protein stores, promote wound healing, prevent infection associated with surgery and immunosuppression, and prevent complications from electrolyte imbalance.

[†] **Chronic phase:** After 1–2 months of receiving the transplant. Goals are to achieve and maintain good overall nutritional status and prevent or minimize the side effects of immunosuppressive therapy, including hyperlipidemia, obesity, hypertension, glucose intolerance/diabetes, and bone disease.

Renal Transplant Flowchart

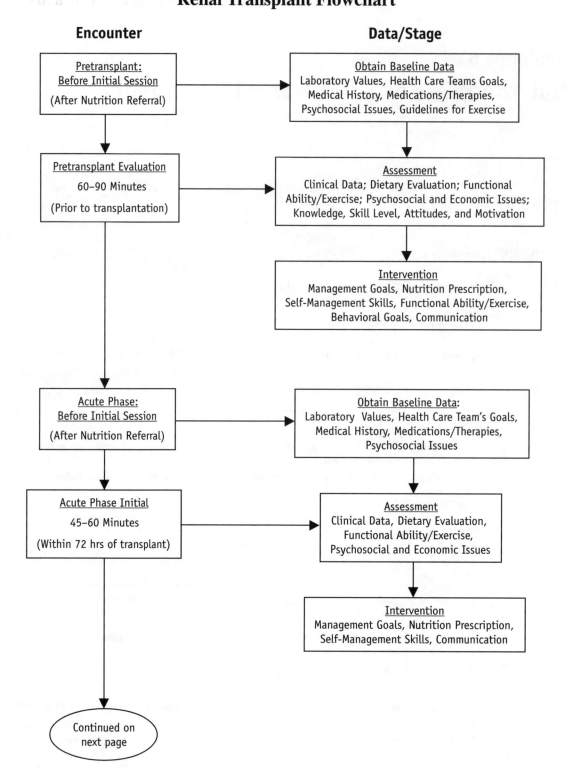

Encounter

Data/Stage

Pretransplant:
Before Initial Session
(After Nutrition Referral)

Obtain Baseline Data
Laboratory Values, Health Care Teams Goals,
Medical History, Medications/Therapies,
Psychosocial Issues, Guidelines for Exercise

Pretransplant Evaluation
60–90 Minutes
(Prior to transplantation)

Assessment
Clinical Data; Dietary Evaluation; Functional
Ability/Exercise; Psychosocial and Economic Issues;
Knowledge, Skill Level, Attitudes, and Motivation

Intervention
Management Goals, Nutrition Prescription,
Self-Management Skills, Functional Ability/Exercise,
Behavioral Goals, Communication

Acute Phase:
Before Initial Session
(After Nutrition Referral)

Obtain Baseline Data:
Laboratory Values, Health Care Team's Goals,
Medical History, Medications/Therapies,
Psychosocial Issues

Acute Phase Initial
45–60 Minutes
(Within 72 hrs of transplant)

Assessment
Clinical Data, Dietary Evaluation,
Functional Ability/Exercise,
Psychosocial and Economic Issues

Intervention
Management Goals, Nutrition Prescription,
Self-Management Skills, Communication

Continued on
next page

Renal Transplant Flowchart (continued)

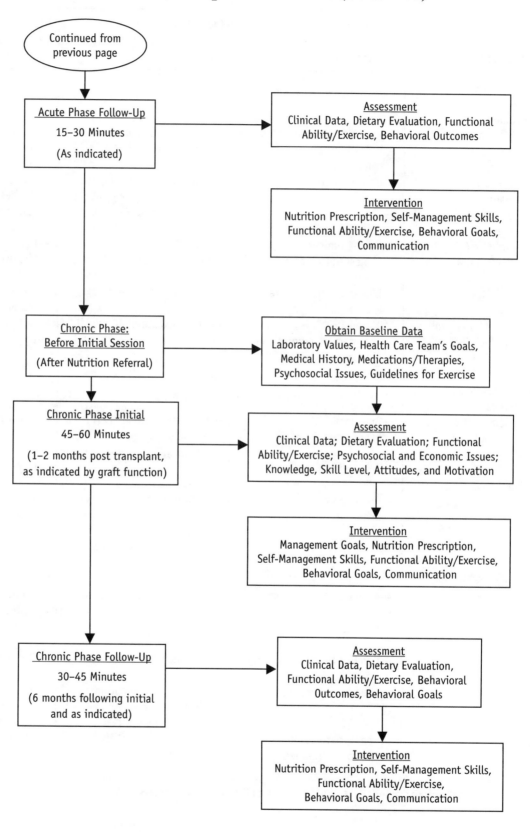

Continued from previous page

Acute Phase Follow-Up
15–30 Minutes
(As indicated)

Assessment
Clinical Data, Dietary Evaluation, Functional Ability/Exercise, Behavioral Outcomes

Intervention
Nutrition Prescription, Self-Management Skills, Functional Ability/Exercise, Behavioral Goals, Communication

Chronic Phase:
Before Initial Session
(After Nutrition Referral)

Obtain Baseline Data
Laboratory Values, Health Care Team's Goals, Medical History, Medications/Therapies, Psychosocial Issues, Guidelines for Exercise

Chronic Phase Initial
45–60 Minutes
(1–2 months post transplant, as indicated by graft function)

Assessment
Clinical Data; Dietary Evaluation; Functional Ability/Exercise; Psychosocial and Economic Issues; Knowledge, Skill Level, Attitudes, and Motivation

Intervention
Management Goals, Nutrition Prescription, Self-Management Skills, Functional Ability/Exercise, Behavioral Goals, Communication

Chronic Phase Follow-Up
30–45 Minutes
(6 months following initial and as indicated)

Assessment
Clinical Data, Dietary Evaluation, Functional Ability/Exercise, Behavioral Outcomes, Behavioral Goals

Intervention
Nutrition Prescription, Self-Management Skills, Functional Ability/Exercise, Behavioral Goals, Communication

Expected Outcomes of Medical Nutrition Therapy

Outcome Assessment Factors	Expected Outcome of Therapy	Ideal/Goal Value Acute Posttransplant Phase*	Ideal/Goal Value Chronic Posttransplant Phase*
Clinical Outcomes • Biochemical Parameters —Albumin —Potassium —Phosphorus —Calcium —Magnesium —Serum glucose (casual) —HgbA1c (diabetes) —Cholesterol —LDL Cholesterol —HDL Cholesterol —Triglycerides (fasting)	—Albumin increasing to 3.5 —Potassium, phosphorus, calcium, magnesium within normal limits —Blood sugar levels within normal limits —Cholesterol progressing toward goal range —LDL and HDL cholesterol within goal ranges —Triglycerides progressing toward goal range	—Albumin 3.5 g/dL —Potassium 3.5–5.0 mEq/L —Phosphorus 2.5–5.0 mg/dL —Calcium 8.5–10.5 mg/dL —Magnesium 1.5–2.0 mEq/L —Serum glucose 80–200 mg/dL —HgbA1c < 7% —Cholesterol 150–200 mg/dL —LDL cholesterol per risk factors (see Appendix H) —HDL cholesterol 40 mg/dL —Triglycerides < 150 mg/dL	—Albumin 3.5–5.0 g/dL —Potassium 3.5–5.0 mEq/L —Phosphorus 2.5–5.0 mg/dL —Calcium 8.5–10.5 mg/dL —Magnesium 1.5–2.0 mEq/L —Serum glucose 80–200 mg/dL —HgbA1c < 7% —Cholesterol 150–200 mg/dL —LDL cholesterol per risk factors (see Appendix H) < —HDL cholesterol 40 mg/dL —Triglycerides < 150 mg/dL
• Hematological Parameters —Hematocrit/ hemoglobin	—Adequate erythropoiesis maintained	—Hematocrit 36–45% (F), 38–50% (M) hemoglobin 12–16 g/dL (F), 14–18 g/dL (M)	—Hematocrit 36–45% (F), 38–50% (M) hemoglobin 12–16 g/dL (F), 14–18 g/dL (M)
• Anthropometrics —Weight	—Reasonable weight achieved/ maintained	—Within reasonable body weight (BMI 20–25) —Weight loss or inappropriate weight gain prevented	—Within reasonable body weight (BMI 20–25) —Inappropriate weight gain prevented
• Clinical Signs and Symptoms	—Adequate body mass maintained —Acceptable level of fat stores achieved/maintained —Level of functional ability maintained —Good appetite maintained —Appropriate blood pressure control maintained	—Adequate muscle/fat stores —Optimum functional ability —Minimum GI symptoms —Food intake > 80% recommended intake —Blood pressure within appropriate limits	—Appropriate muscle/fat stores —Optimum functional ability —Minimum GI symptoms —Food intake > 80% recommended intake —Blood pressure within appropriate limits

*For pretransplant goals, see Guideline 2, Adult Dialysis Patients

Continued

Expected Outcomes of Medical Nutrition Therapy (continued)

Outcome Assessment Factors	Expected Outcome of Therapy	Ideal/Goal Value Acute Posttransplant Phase*	Ideal/Goal Value Chronic Posttransplant Phase*
Patient/Caregiver Behavioral Outcomes • Food selection/meal planning • Nutrient needs • Potential food/drug interactions • Exercise	—Exhibits positive changes in food selection and amounts. —If diabetic, times meals and snacks appropriately. —Identifies foods high in calories, protein, simple sugars, fat, cholesterol, and sodium. —Maintains adequate fluid intake. —Verbalizes potential food/drug interactions. —If no medical limitations, gradually increases or continues physical activity level.	**MNT Goals** 1. Makes appropriate food choices and takes medications as prescribed. 2. Maintains adequate calorie and protein intake. 3. Adjusts intake per short-term complications (e.g., transient hyperglycemia, transient hyperkalemia). 4. Maintains adequate fluid intake. 5. Maintains lab values within acceptable limits. 6. If diabetic, maintains stable glucose levels through appropriate dietary practices. 7. If no medical limitations, initiation of an exercise program.	**MNT Goals** 1. Makes appropriate food choices and takes medications as prescribed. 2. Adjusts intake of calories, protein, simple sugars, fat, cholesterol, and sodium to minimize risk of weight gain, hyperglycemia, hyperlipidemia, hypertension. 3. Maintains adequate fluid intake. 4. Maintains lab values within acceptable limits. 5. If diabetic, maintains stable glucose levels through appropriate dietary practices. 6. If no medical limitations, maintenance of an exercise program.

Pretransplant Evaluation: Minimum Baseline Data Needed for Medical Nutrition Therapy

Factor	Data Needed
Laboratory Values with Dates (within 30 days of session)	1. BUN, creatinine 2. Albumin 3. Sodium, potassium, phosphorus, calcium 4. Serum glucose 5. Lipid profile 6. Serum bicarbonate 7. PTH, alkaline phosphatase 8. Hematocrit/hemoglobin 9. Dialysis adequacy, PET results, if available 10. Urinalysis results (e.g., volume, urea, protein), if available 11. Others as appropriate (e.g., ferritin, transferrin saturation, glycosylated hemoglobin, vitamin B12, folate)
Health Care Team's Goals for Patient	1. Patient prognosis 2. Expected outcome of nutrition therapy 3. Expected date of transplant, if available
Medical History	1. Disease/condition causing renal failure 2. History of renal disease and treatment 3. Concurrent medical conditions (e.g., diabetes, cardiovascular disease, GI problems, hypertension, hyperlipidemia) 4. Any other medical or physical conditions with potential nutritional implications (e.g., surgery, infection, CVA, blindness, neuropathies)
Medications/Therapies	1. Current treatment mode for ESRD 2. Type of dialysis therapy and prescription, if appropriate 3. Diet order, tube-feeding order, parenteral nutrition order, and/or IDPN/IPN order 4. Any other treatments or therapies that may affect nutritional intake or status 5. Antihypertensives, diuretics 6. Anticoagulants 7. Phosphate binders 8. Vitamin/mineral supplements 9. Any other medications with food/drug interactions or nutritional impact (e.g., diabetes medications, GI medications, lipid-lowering medications, steroids, hormonal replacement)
Psychosocial Issues	1. Learning disabilities 2. Vision, hearing abilities 3. Cultural or language barriers 4. Mental status
Guidelines for Exercise	1. Medical clearance for exercise 2. Exercise limitations, if any

Pretransplant Nutrition Assessment

Session: *Pretransplant Evaluation*   Length: *60–90 minutes*   Time: *Prior to transplantation*

Factor	Assessments
Clinical Data	1. Review Pretransplant Evaluation: Minimum Baseline Data. 2. Obtain current height, dry weight, and BMI. 3. Obtain weight history, recent weight changes, and weight goals. 4. Determine IBW and/or UBW adjusted for amputation or obesity, and percentage IBW and/or percentage UBW (see Appendix B). 5. Assess muscle and fat stores, presence of edema. 6. Assess for physical signs of nutrient deficiencies/excesses or increased needs (e.g., decubiti, poor wound healing, thinning hair, pale conjunctiva, cheilosis). 7. Determine nitrogen balance using urea kinetics, if appropriate (see Appendix D). 8. Assess blood pressure control.
Dietary Evaluation	1. Determine previous dietary instruction and practices. 2. Determine usual food intake and pattern of intake. 3. Assess appetite, GI issues, tolerance of oral intake, and food allergies/intolerances. 4. Assess feeding issues (e.g., chewing, swallowing). 5. Determine use of vitamin/mineral, herbal, or other nutrition supplements. 6. Determine alcohol/drug/tobacco use and history. 7. For PD, determine glucose absorption and calories from dialysate (see Appendix C). 8. Assess intake of calories, protein, sodium, potassium, phosphorus, calcium, fluids, and other nutrients as indicated. 9. Assess diet order, tube-feeding order, parenteral nutrition order, and/or IDPN/IPN order for appropriateness.
Functional Ability/Exercise	1. Determine level of functional ability and recent changes. 2. Assess ability to feed self and needs for assistance. 3. Determine activity level and exercise habits. 4. Determine physical or motivational limitations to exercise.
Psychosocial and Economic Issues	1. Assess living situation, cooking facilities, finances, educational background, employment, literacy, and other factors that may affect availability of food. 2. Assess ethnic or religious belief considerations. 3. Assess availability of support systems. 4. Determine if other relevant psychosocial or economic issues exist.
Knowledge, Skill Level, Attitudes, and Motivation	1. Assess basic knowledge level of dietary guidelines for the patient's mode of treatment. 2. Assess attitudes toward nutrition and health and adherence with current dietary prescription and regimen. 3. Determine patient's willingness and ability to learn and make appropriate changes.

Pretransplant Nutrition Intervention

Session: *Pretransplant Evaluation*   Length: *60–90 minutes*   Time: *Prior to transplantation*

Factor	Interventions
Management Goals	1. Identify management goals of health care team. 2. Identify patient goals and expectations.
Nutrition Prescription	1. Calories—individualized; sufficient calories to achieve and maintain appropriate weight and body stores 2. Protein—individualized; sufficient protein to maintain or replete protein stores prior to surgery. May require supplementation. 3. Fats—for lipid abnormalities: fats, cholesterol, and carbohydrates adjusted per severity of risk factors (see Appendixes G and H) 4. Sodium/potassium—as indicated by mode of treatment of ESRD 5. Phosphorus/calcium—individualized; as indicated by laboratory values and mode of treatment of ESRD to reduce risk of bone disease 6. Fluids—as indicated by mode of treatment of ESRD 7. Vitamin/mineral supplementation—as indicated by mode of treatment of ESRD
Self-Management Skills	1. Discuss simple definitions and examples of calories, protein, and other nutrients as appropriate (e.g., fats, sodium, potassium, phosphorus, calcium). 2. Discuss importance of adequate nutrition prior to surgery and specific dietary needs to reduce risk of infection and promote wound healing. 3. If patient clinically obese, encourage patient to decrease fat weight to minimize surgical risk and postoperative complications. 4. If hyperlipidemic, discuss cholesterol and saturated fat and methods for reducing dietary fat and cholesterol. 5. Discuss role and effect of diet and medications in renal disease and transplantation. 6. Discuss long-term dietary therapy and MNT goals for transplantation (e.g., reduce cardiovascular risk and risk of bone disease). 7. Assess comprehension of education provided and projected compliance.
Functional Ability/Exercise	1. Provide necessary referrals for assistance with self-feeding and other activities of daily living (e.g., OT, PT, speech therapy). 2. Discuss exercise recommendations, if appropriate.
Behavioral Goals	1. Address eating and exercise behaviors. 2. Identify and summarize short-term behavioral goals that are specific and achievable. 3. Establish follow-up plan, if appropriate.
Communication	1. Document current nutritional status, plan of care, and goals of medical nutrition therapy. 2. Report recommendations/concerns to appropriate health care team member (e.g., MD, RN, pharmacist, social worker). 3. Provide information regarding nutrition prescription and dietary guidelines to dialysis facility, extended-care facility, home health care facilities, if appropriate.

Acute Phase Evaluation: Minimum Baseline Data Needed for Medical Nutrition Therapy

Factor	Data Needed
Laboratory Values with Dates	1. BUN, creatinine 2. Albumin 3. Sodium, potassium 4. Phosphorus, calcium, magnesium 5. Serum glucose 6. Lipid profile 7. PTH 8. Hematocrit/hemoglobin 9. Others as appropriate (e.g., ferritin, glycosylated hemoglobin)
Health Care Team's Goals for Patient	1. Patient prognosis 2. Expected outcome of nutrition therapy
Medical History	1. Disease/condition causing renal failure 2. History of renal disease and treatment prior to transplant 3. Current functional status of graft 4. Concurrent medical conditions (e.g., diabetes, cardiovascular disease, GI problems, hypertension, hyperlipidemia) 5. Any other medical or physical conditions with potential nutritional implications (e.g., surgery, infection, CVA, blindness, neuropathies)
Medications/Therapies	1. Type of dialysis therapy and prescription, if appropriate 2. Diet order, tube-feeding order, and/or parenteral nutrition order 3. IV administration 4. Any other therapies/treatments that may affect nutritional intake or status 5. Immunosuppressants 6. Antihypertensives, diuretics 7. Vitamin/mineral supplements 8. Any other medications with food/drug interactions or nutritional impact (e.g., diabetes medications, GI medications, lipid-lowering medications, hormonal replacement)
Psychosocial Issues (as appropriate)	1. Learning disabilities 2. Vision, hearing abilities 3. Cultural or language barriers 4. Mental status

Initial Nutrition Assessment: Acute Phase

Session: *Acute Phase Initial*   Length: *45–60 minutes*   Time: *Within 72 hours of transplant*

Factor	Assessments
Clinical Data	1. Review Acute Phase Evaluation: Minimum Baseline Data. 2. Obtain current height, weight, estimated dry weight, and BMI. 3. Obtain weight history, recent weight changes, and weight goals. 4. Determine IBW and/or UBW adjusted for amputation or obesity, and percentage IBW and/or percentage UBW (see Appendix B). 5. Assess muscle and fat stores, presence of edema. 6. Assess for physical signs of nutrient deficiencies/excesses or increased needs (e.g., decubiti, poor wound healing, thinning hair, pale conjunctiva, cheilosis).
Dietary Evaluation	1. Determine usual food intake and pattern of intake prior to admission. 2. Assess appetite, GI issues, tolerance of oral intake, and food allergies/intolerances. 3. Assess feeding issues (e.g., chewing, swallowing). 4. Determine use of vitamin/mineral, herbal, or other nutrition supplements. 5. Determine alcohol/drug/tobacco use and history. 6. Determine hydration status and assess fluid intake/output. 7. Assess intake of calories, protein, sodium, potassium, phosphorus, calcium and other nutrients as indicated. 8. Assess diet order, tube-feeding order, and/or parenteral nutrition order for appropriateness.
Functional Ability/Exercise	1. Determine level of functional ability and recent changes in ability. 2. Assess ability to feed self and needs for assistance.
Psychosocial and Economic Issues	1. Assess educational background, literacy level, as appropriate. 2. Assess ethnic or religious belief considerations. 3. Assess availability of support systems. 4. Determine whether other relevant psychosocial or economic issues exist.

Initial Nutrition Intervention: Acute Phase

Session: *Acute Phase Initial*   Length: *45–60 minutes*   Time: *Within 72 hours of transplant*

Factor	Interventions
Management Goals	1. Identify management goals of health care team. 2. Identify patient goals and expectations.
Nutrition Prescription	1. Calories—individualized; 30–35 kcal/kg; (adjust for nitrogen balance, if available) 2. Protein = 1.3–1.5 g/kg IBW; may be higher depending on stress, metabolic needs, or corticosteroid dose 3. Carbohydrates—50–60% of total calories; may need to limit for hyperglycemia 4. Fat—to provide additional calories as needed; emphasize PUFA and MUFA 5. Sodium—individualized; approximately 2–4 g/day 6. Potassium—restricted to 2–4 g/day if hyperkalemic 7. Phosphorus—individualized per laboratory results; may require supplementation or restriction 8. Calcium—individualized per laboratory results; approximately 800–1500 mg/day; may require supplementation 9. Magnesium—individualized, may require supplementation 10. Fluids—as desired; limited only by graft function 11. Vitamin/mineral supplementation as appropriate; US RDA
Self-Management Skills	1. Discuss nutrition therapy recommendations with patient and/or caregiver. 2. Discuss basic dietary guidelines for transplant acute phase as indicated and reinforce temporary nature of dietary recommendations as based on medical condition and laboratory results. 3. Discuss role and effect of diet and medications in transplantation, if appropriate. 4. Assess comprehension of education provided and projected outcome.
Functional Ability	1. Provide necessary referrals for assistance with self-feeding and other activities of daily living (e.g., OT, PT, speech therapy).
Communication	1. Document current nutritional status, plan of care, and goals of MNT. 2. Report recommendations/concerns to appropriate health care team member (e.g., MD, RN, pharmacist, social worker).

Follow-up Nutrition Assessment: Acute Phase

Session: *Acute Follow-up*   Length: *15–30 minutes*   Time: *As indicated*

Factor	Assessments
Clinical Data	1. Review changes in medical status and recent/planned therapies (e.g., medications, dialysis, surgery). 2. Obtain current functional status of graft. 3. Review any new or updated laboratory data. 4. Assess changes in weight and presence of edema. 5. Assess for physical signs of nutrient deficiencies/excesses or increased needs (e.g., decubiti, poor wound healing, thinning hair, pale conjunctiva, cheilosis). 6. Assess blood pressure control. 7. Assess effectiveness of previous nutrition intervention.
Dietary Evaluation	1. Determine current GI or feeding issues or concerns, tolerance of oral intake. 2. Assess changes in patient's food intake and/or appetite. 3. Determine fluid intake/output and hydration status. 4. Assess dietary intake and/or nutritional support intake for adequacy and appropriateness.
Functional Ability/Exercise	1. Assess changes in functional ability. 2. Assess changes in activity level.
Behavioral Outcomes	1. Assess understanding of nutrition therapy recommendations. 2. Assess understanding of basic dietary guidelines for transplant acute phase. 3. Assess understanding of role and effect of diet and medications in transplantation.

Follow-up Nutrition Intervention: Acute Phase

Session: *Acute Follow-up*   Length: *15–30 minutes*   Time: *As indicated*

Factor	Interventions
Nutrition Prescription (as appropriate)	1. Provide feedback on laboratory results, blood pressure control, changes in weight. 2. Provide feedback on food/meal plan, food choices, and portions. 3. Recommend changes in nutrient intake amounts or habits that can improve outcomes. 4. Adjust MNT.
Self-Management Skills (as appropriate)	1. Discuss nutrition therapy changes and recommendations with patient and/or caregiver as indicated. 2. Discuss simple definitions of calories, protein, carbohydrates, fats, and other nutrients as indicated. 3. Discuss risk of weight gain posttransplant and health risks associated with obesity. 4. Discuss risk of hyperlipidemia posttransplant and associated health risks. 5. Discuss potential for hyperglycemia based on blood glucose or high dose steroids, family history, and weight. 6. For diagnosed diabetes, discuss basic dietary guidelines and timing of meals and snacks, if indicated. 7. Discuss food/drug interactions as indicated. 8. Discuss nutritional implications of medications. 9. Assess comprehension of education provided and projected compliance.
Functional Ability/Exercise	1. Refer to OT, PT, speech therapy as appropriate. 2. Encourage regular exercise per tolerance to minimize muscle wasting and bone loss.
Behavioral Goals	1. Identify and summarize short-term behavioral goals that are specific and achievable. 2. Establish follow-up plan.
Communication	1. Document current nutritional status, plan of care, and goals of MNT. 2. Report recommendations/concerns to appropriate health care team member (e.g., MD, RN, pharmacist, social worker).

Chronic Phase Evaluation: Minimum Baseline Data Needed for Medical Nutrition Therapy

Factor	Data Needed
Laboratory Values with Dates	1. BUN, creatinine 2. Albumin 3. Sodium, potassium 4. Phosphorus, calcium, magnesium 5. Serum glucose 6. Lipid profile 7. PTH, alkaline phosphatase 8. Hematocrit, hemoglobin 9. Others as appropriate (e.g., ferritin, glycosylated hemoglobin)
Health Care Team's Goals for Patient	1. Patient prognosis 2. Expected outcomes of nutrition therapy
Medical History	1. Disease/condition causing renal failure 2. History of renal disease and treatment 3. Current status of graft function 4. Concurrent medical conditions (e.g., diabetes, cancer, HIV, cardiovascular disease, GI problems, hypertension, hyperlipidemia) 5. Any other medical or physical conditions with potential nutritional implications (e.g., surgery, infection, CVA, chemotherapy, blindness, neuropathies)
Medications/Therapies	1. Diet order, tube-feeding order, and/or parenteral nutrition order 2. Any other therapies/treatments that may affect nutritional intake or status 3. Immunosuppressants 4. Antihypertensives, diuretics 5. Vitamin/mineral supplements 6. Any other medications with food/drug interactions or nutritional impact (e.g., diabetes medications, GI medications, lipid-lowering medications, hormonal replacement)
Psychosocial Issues	1. Learning disabilities 2. Vision, hearing abilities 3. Cultural or language barriers 4. Mental status
Guidelines for Exercise	1. Medical clearance for exercise, if appropriate 2. Exercise limitations, if any

Initial Nutrition Assessment: Chronic Phase

Session: *Chronic Phase Initial* Length: *45–60 minutes* Time: *1–2 months post transplant,*
as indicated by graft function

Factor	Assessments
Clinical Data	1. Review Chronic Phase Evaluation: Minimum Baseline Data. 2. Obtain current height, weight, and BMI. 3. Obtain weight history, recent weight changes, and weight goals. 4. Determine IBW and/or UBW adjusted for amputation or obesity, and percentage IBW and/or percentage UBW (see Appendix B). 5. Assess muscle and fat stores, presence of edema. 6. Assess for physical signs of nutrient deficiencies/excesses or increased needs (e.g., decubiti, poor wound healing, thinning hair, pale conjunctiva, cheilosis). 7. Assess blood pressure control.
Dietary Evaluation	1. Determine previous dietary instruction and practices. 2. Determine usual food intake and pattern of intake. 3. Assess appetite, GI issues, tolerance of oral intake, and food allergies/intolerances. 4. Assess feeding issues (e.g., chewing, swallowing). 5. Determine use of vitamin/mineral, herbal, or other nutrition supplements. 6. Assess alcohol/drug/tobacco use and history. 7. Assess intake of calories, protein, carbohydrate, fat, sodium, potassium, phosphorus, calcium and other nutrients as indicated. 8. Assess diet order, tube-feeding order, and/or parenteral nutrition order for appropriateness.
Functional Ability/Exercise	1. Determine level of functional ability and recent changes. 2. Assess ability to feed self and needs for assistance. 3. Determine activity level and exercise habits. 4. Determine physical or motivational limitations to exercise.
Psychosocial and Economic Issues	1. Assess living situation, cooking facilities, finances, educational background, employment, literacy, and other factors that may affect availability of food. 2. Assess ethnic or religious belief considerations. 3. Assess availability of support systems. 4. Determine if other relevant psychosocial or economic issues exist.
Knowledge, Skill Level, Attitudes, and Motivation	1. Assess basic knowledge level of dietary guidelines for transplant patients. 2. Assess basic knowledge level of impact of transplant therapy on nutrition. 3. Assess attitudes toward nutrition and health. 4. Determine patient's willingness and ability to learn and make appropriate changes.

Initial Nutrition Intervention: Chronic Phase

Session: *Chronic Phase Initial*   Length: *45–60 minutes*   Time: *1–2 months post transplant,*
as indicated by graft function

Factor	Interventions
Management Goals	1. Identify management goals of health care team. 2. Identify patient goals and expectations.
Nutrition Prescription	1. Calories—individualized; to achieve/maintain desirable body weight 2. Protein = 1.0–1.2 g/kg IBW; limit with chronic rejection 3. Carbohydrates—50–60% total calories; limit concentrated sweets and emphasize complex carbohydrates 4. Fats—fats and cholesterol per National Cholesterol Education Program guidelines and severity of risk factors (see Appendixes G and H) 5. Sodium—individualized; appx. 2–4 g/day 6. Potassium—restrict to 2–4 g/day if hyperkalemic 7. Phosphorus—restrict or supplement as needed 8. Calcium—800–1500 mg/day 9. Fluids—as desired 10. Vitamin/mineral supplementation as appropriate; US RDA
Self-Management Skills	1. Discuss simple definitions and examples of calories, protein, carbohydrates, fats and other nutrients as appropriate (e.g., sodium, potassium, phosphorus, calcium). 2. Discuss dietary guidelines to reduce risk of rejection, cardiovascular disease, diabetes, and osteoporosis. 3. For diabetes, discuss basic dietary guidelines and timing of meals and snacks, if indicated. 4. Discuss appropriate weight and weight goals post transplant, risk of weight gain post transplant, health risks associated with obesity, and measures to prevent inappropriate weight gain. 5. Discuss use and effect of vitamin supplements. 6. Discuss food/drug interactions as indicated. 7. Discuss role and effect of diet and medications in transplantation. 8. Assess comprehension of education provided and projected compliance.
Functional Ability/Exercise	1. Provide necessary referrals for assistance with self-feeding and other activities of daily living (e.g., OT, PT, speech therapy). 2. Discuss exercise recommendations, if appropriate.
Behavioral Goals	1. Address eating and exercise behaviors. 2. Identify and summarize short-term behavioral goals that are specific and achievable. 3. Establish follow-up plan.
Communication	1. Document current nutritional status, plan of care, and goals of medical nutrition therapy. 2. Report recommendations/concerns to appropriate health care team member (e.g., MD, RN, pharmacist, social worker). 3. Provide information regarding nutrition prescription and dietary guidelines to extended-care facility, home health care facilities, if appropriate.

Follow-up Nutrition Assessment: Chronic Phase

Session: *Chronic Follow-up*   Length: *30–45 minutes*   Time: *6 months following initial and as indicated*

Factor	Assessments
Clinical Data	1. Review changes in medical status and recent/planned therapies (e.g., medications, surgery). 2. Review recent laboratory data. 3. Assess changes in weight. 4. Determine BMI, IBW and/or UBW adjusted for amputation or obesity, and percentage IBW and/or percentage UBW (see Appendix B). 5. Assess muscle and fat stores, presence of edema. 6. Assess for physical signs of nutrient deficiencies/excesses or increased needs (e.g., decubiti, poor wound healing, thinning hair, pale conjunctiva, cheilosis). 7. Assess blood pressure control. 8. Assess effectiveness of previous nutrition intervention.
Dietary Evaluation	1. Determine current GI or feeding issues or concerns, tolerance of oral intake. 2. Assess changes in patient's food intake and/or appetite. 3. Determine use of vitamin/mineral, herbal, or other nutrition supplements. 4. Assess intake of calories, protein, carbohydrate, fat, sodium, potassium, phosphorus, and calcium or other nutrients as indicated for appropriateness. 5. Assess diet order, tube-feeding order, and/or parenteral nutrition order for appropriateness.
Functional Ability/Exercise	1. Determine level of functional ability and recent changes. 2. Assess ability to feed self and needs for assistance. 3. Assess changes in activity level or exercise habits. 4. Determine physical or motivational limitations to exercise.
Psychosocial and Economic Issues	1. Assess changes in living situation, cooking facilities, finances, education, employment, literacy, and other factors that may affect availability of food. 2. Assess availability of support systems. 3. Determine if other relevant psychosocial or economic issues exist.
Behavioral Outcomes	1. Assess understanding of simple definitions and examples of calories, protein, carbohydrates, fats and other nutrients as appropriate (e.g., sodium, potassium, phosphorus, calcium). 2. Assess understanding of dietary guidelines to reduce risk of rejection, cardiovascular disease, diabetes, and osteoporosis. 3. For diabetes, assess understanding of basic dietary guidelines and timing of meals and snacks. 4. Assess understanding of appropriate weight and weight goals post transplant, health risks associated with obesity, and measures to prevent inappropriate weight gain. 5. Assess understanding of use and effect of vitamin supplements. 6. Assess understanding of food/drug interactions. 7. Assess understanding of role and effect of diet and medications in transplantation. 8. Determine further improvements that can be made in the quality of the diet.
Behavioral Goals	1. Assess achievement of prior behavioral goals. 2. Determine willingness and ability to make further changes.

Follow-up Nutrition Intervention: Chronic Phase

Session: *Chronic Follow-up*   Length: *30–45 minutes*   Time: *6 months following initial and as indicated*

Factor	Interventions
Management Goals	1. Reassess and adjust management goals of patient and health care team.
Nutrition Prescription	1. Provide feedback on lab results, blood pressure control, changes in weight. 2. Provide feedback on food/meal plan, food choices, and portions. 3. Recommend changes in nutrient intake or habits that may improve outcomes. 4. Adjust MNT as appropriate.
Self-Management Skills	1. Review and reinforce self-management skills from prior session. 2. Provide and review educational materials as appropriate. 3. If medication change, discuss potential food/drug interaction and impact in transplantation. 4. Assess comprehension of education provided and projected compliance.
Functional Ability/Exercise	1. Provide necessary referrals for assistance with self-feeding and other activities of daily living (e.g., OT, PT, speech therapy). 2. Discuss changes in exercise recommendations if appropriate.
Behavioral Goals	1. Reset short-term behavioral goals that are specific and achievable. 2. Review and reinforce long term goals. 3. Establish follow-up plan.
Communication	1. Document current nutritional status, plan of care, and goals of medical nutrition therapy. 2. Report recommendations/concerns to appropriate health care team member (e.g., MD, RN, pharmacist, social worker). 3. Provide information regarding nutrition prescription and dietary guidelines to extended-care facility, home health care facilities, if appropriate.

Bibliography

American Diabetes Association Position Statement: Standards of Medical Care for Patients with Diabetes Mellitus. *Diabetes Care.* 1997;20(Suppl 1):S5–S13.

American Diabetes Association. *Maximizing the Role of Nutrition in Diabetes Management.* Alexandria, Va: American Diabetes Association, Inc.; 1994.

Andress DL. Treatment of low turnover bone disease in renal failure. *Nephrol Exchange.* 1996;6(1): 16–20.

Arnadottir M, Berg AL. Treatment of hyperlipidemia in renal transplant recipients. *Transplantation.* 1997;63(3):339–345.

Beto JA. Which diet for which renal failure: Making sense of the options. *J Am Diet Assoc.* 1995;95(8):898–903.

Blue LS. Nutrition considerations in kidney transplantation. *Top Clin Nutr.* 1992;7(3):17–23.

Borges W, Gonzalez Caraballo Z, Santiago Delphin EA, Morales Otero L. Chronic effect of a high-protein low-fat diet in transplant patients. *Transplant Proc.* 1996;8(6):3400–3401.

Byham Gray L. Nutritional implications of renal transplantation, Part II. *Renal Nutr Forum.* 1994;13(1):1–3.

Byham Gray L. Nutritional implications of renal transplantation. *Renal Nutr Forum.* 1993;12(4): 1–3.

Cappuccio FP, MacGregor GA. Dietary salt restriction: benefits for cardiovascular disease and beyond. *Curr Opin Nephrol Hypertens.* 1997;6:477–482.

The Chicago Dietetic Association and The South Suburban Dietetic Association. *Manual of Clinical Dietetics.* 5th ed. Chicago, Ill: The American Dietetic Association; 1996.

Dimeny E, Tufveson G, Lithell H, Larsson E, Siegbahn A, Fellstrom B. The influence of pretransplant lipoprotein abnormalities on the early results of renal transplantation. *Eur J Clin Invest.* 1993;23:572–579.

Divakar D, Bailey RR, Price M, Frampton C, George PM. Effect of diet on posttransplant hyperlipidaemia. *NZ Med J.* 1992;105:79–80.

Farkas-Hirsch R, ed. *Intensive Diabetes Management.* Alexandria, Va: American Diabetes Association; 1995.

Gottschlich MM, Matarese LE, Shronts EP, eds. *Nutrition Support Dietetics Core Curriculum.* 2nd ed. Silver Spring, Md: American Society of Parenteral Enteral Nutrition; 1993.

Grant A, DeHoog S. *Nutritional Assessment and Support.* 4th ed. Seattle, Wash: Anne Grant/Susan DeHoog; 1991.

Hasse J. Nutritional management of renal transplant patients. *Diet Curr.* 1993;20(5):21–24.

Hirschberg RR, Kopple JD. Energy requirements in patients with renal failure. *Contrib Nephrol.* 1990;81:124–135.

Horber FF, Zurcher RM, Herren H, Crivelli MA, Robotti G, Frey FJ. Altered body fat distribution in Patients with glucocorticoid treatment and in patients on long-term dialysis. *Am J Clin Nutr.* 1986;43:758–769.

Jaggers HJ, Allman MA, Chan M. Changes in clinical profile and dietary considerations after renal transplantation. *J Renal Nutr.* 1996;6(1):12–20.

Jindal RM. Post-transplant hyperlipidemia. *Postgrad Med J.* 1997;73:785–793.

Johnson CP, Gallagher-Lepak S, Zhu Y, Porth C, Kelber S, Roza AM, Adams MB. Factors influencing weight gain after renal transplantation. *Transplantation.* 1993;56(4):822–827.

Kaiske BL. Risk factors for cardiovascular disease after renal transplantation. *Miner Electrolyte Metab.* 1993;19:186–195.

Kasiske BL. Hyperlipidemia in patients with chronic renal disease. *Am J Kidney Dis.* 1998;32(5, Suppl 3):S142–S156.

Lebovitz HE, ed. *Therapy for Diabetes Mellitus and Related Disorders.* 2nd ed. Alexandria, Va: American Diabetes Association, Inc.; 1994.

Levey AS. Controlling the epidemic of cardiovascular disease in chronic renal disease: Where do we start? *Am J Kidney Dis.* 1998;32(5,Suppl 3):S5–S13.

Levine DZ, ed. *Care of the Renal Patient.* 2nd ed. Philadelphia, Pa: W.B. Saunders Company; 1991.

Mailloux LU, Levey AS. Hypertension in patients with chronic renal disease. *Am J Kidney Dis.* 1998;32(5,Suppl 3):S120–S141.

Manske CL. Hyperglycemia and intensive glycemic control in diabetic patients with chronic renal disease. *Am J Kidney Dis.* 1998;32(5,Suppl 3):S157–S171.

Marine-Brundage KA, Kasiske BL. Nutritional Management of Renal Transplantation. In Kopple JD, Massry SG, eds. *Nutritional Management of Renal Disease.* Baltimore, Md: Williams & Wilkins; 1997.

Markell MS, Armenti V, Danovitch G, Sumrani N. Hyperlipidemia and glucose intolerance in the post-renal transplant patient. *J Am Soc Nephrol.* 1994;4:S37–S47.

Massy ZA, Kasiske BL. Post-transplant hyperlipidemia: mechanisms and management. *J Am Soc Nephrol.* 1996;7:971–977.

Mathieu RL, Casez JP, Jaeger P, Montandon A, Peheim E, Horber FF. Altered body composition and fuel metabolism in stable kidney transplant patients on immuno-suppressive monotherapy with cyclosporine A. *Eur J Clin Invest.* 1994;24:195–200.

Miller DG, Levine SE, D'Elia JA, Bistrian BR. Nutritional status of diabetic and nondiabetic patients after renal transplantation. *Am J Clin Nutr.* 1986;44:66–69.

Moe SM. The treatment of steroid-induced bone loss in transplantation. *Curr Opin Nephrol Hypertens.* 1997;6:544–549.

Moore LW, Osama Gaber A. Patterns of early weight change after renal transplantation. *J Renal Nutr.* 1996;6(1):21–25.

Moore RA, Callahan MF, Cody M, Adams PL, Litchford M, Buckner K, Galloway J. The effect of the American Heart Association Step One Diet on hyperlipidemia following renal transplantation. *Transplantation.* 1990;49(1):60–62.

Oda H, Keane WF. Lipid Abnormalities in end stage renal disease. *Nephrol Dial Transplant.* 1998;13(Suppl 1):45–49.

Ong CS, Pollock CA, Caterson RJ, Mahoney JF, Waugh DA, Ibels LS. Hyperlipidemia in renal transplant recipients: Natural history and response to treatment. *Medicine.* 1994;73(4):215–223.

Pagenkemper JJ, Foulks CJ. Nutritional management of the adult renal transplant patient. *J Renal Nutr.* 1991;1(3):119–124.

Park SB, Kim HC, Lee SH, Cho WH, Park CH. Evolution of serum ferritin levels in renal transplant recipients with severe iron overload. *Transplant Proc.* 1994;26(4):2054–2055.

Perez R. Managing nutrition problems in transplant patients. *Nutr Clin Pract.* 1993;8:28–32.

Rao M, Jacob CK, Shastry JCM. Post-renal transplant diabetes mellitus—A retrospective study. *Nephrol Dial Transplant.* 1992;7:1039–1042.

Stover J, ed. *A Clinical Guide to Nutrition Care in End-Stage Renal Disease.* 2nd ed. Chicago, Ill: The American Dietetic Association; 1994.

Strejc J, Weil S. Nutritional management of the renal transplant recipient. *Clin Strategies: AKF Newsletter for Nephrol Professionals.* 1996;3(2):5–13.

Sullivan SS, Anderson EJ, Best S, Sonnenberg LM, Williams WW. The effect of diet on hypercholesterolemia in renal transplant recipients. *J Renal Nutr.* 1996;6(3):141–151.

Sumrani NB, Delaney V, Ding Z, Davis R, Daskalakis P, Friedman EA, Butt KM, Hong JH.

Diabetes mellitus after renal transplantation in the cyclosporine era—An analysis of risk factors. *Transplantation.* 1991;51(2):343–347.

Torres A, Rodriguez AP, Concepcion MT, Garcia S, Rufino M, Martin B, Perez L, Machado M, de Bonis E, Losada B, Hernandez D, Lorenzo V. Parathyroid function in long-term renal transplant patients: Importance of pre-transplant PTH concentrations. *Nephrol Dial Transplant.* 1998;13(Suppl 3):94–97.

Varella L, Utermohlen V. Nutritional support for the patient with renal failure. *Crit Care Nurs Clin N Amer.* 1993;5(1):79–96.

Von Kiparski A, Frei D, Uhlschmid G, Largiader F, Binswanger U. Post-transplant diabetes mellitus I renal allograft recipients: A matched-pair control study. *Nephrol Dial Transplant.* 1990;5:220–225.

Wenger NK. Lipid metabolism, physical activity, and postmenopausal hormone therapy. *Am J Kidney Dis.* 1998;32(5,Suppl 3):S80–S88.

Wheeler DC. Cardiovascular risk factors in patients with chronic renal failure. *J Renal Nutr.* 1997;7(4):182–186.

Zuercher RM, Koehn S, Theil G, Frey FJ, Horber FF. Preservation of body composition in renal transplant patients by cyclosporin, as opposed to prednisone. *Transplantation.* 1990;50(1):159–162.

Guideline 7
Nutrition Care of Adult Pregnant ESRD Patients

Synopsis/Summary

Diagnosis: Pregnancy in End-Stage Renal Disease (Adult 18+ years)

Exceptions for Chart Audit: Patients who are younger than 18 years of age; patients who transfer to another unit, or die within 1 month. For subjective data, patients who are unwilling or unable to communicate and have no caregivers who wish to do so.

Encounter	Length of Contact	Intervals Between Encounters
Initial	60–90 minutes	Within 1 month of diagnosis of pregnancy
Follow-up Sessions	30–45 minutes	Weekly for dialysis, monthly for transplants and renal insufficiency

End-Stage Renal Disease and Pregnancy Flowchart

Encounter   **Data/Stage**

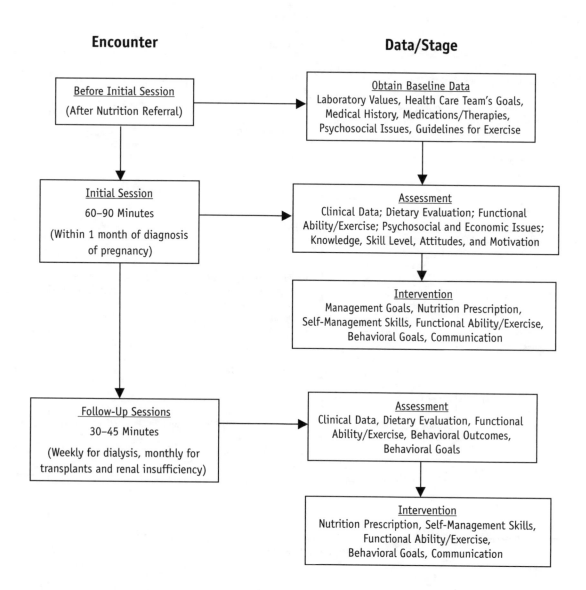

Before Initial Session
(After Nutrition Referral)

Obtain Baseline Data
Laboratory Values, Health Care Team's Goals,
Medical History, Medications/Therapies,
Psychosocial Issues, Guidelines for Exercise

Initial Session
60–90 Minutes
(Within 1 month of diagnosis
of pregnancy)

Assessment
Clinical Data; Dietary Evaluation; Functional
Ability/Exercise; Psychosocial and Economic Issues;
Knowledge, Skill Level, Attitudes, and Motivation

Intervention
Management Goals, Nutrition Prescription,
Self-Management Skills, Functional Ability/Exercise,
Behavioral Goals, Communication

Follow-Up Sessions
30–45 Minutes
(Weekly for dialysis, monthly for
transplants and renal insufficiency)

Assessment
Clinical Data, Dietary Evaluation, Functional
Ability/Exercise, Behavioral Outcomes,
Behavioral Goals

Intervention
Nutrition Prescription, Self-Management Skills,
Functional Ability/Exercise,
Behavioral Goals, Communication

Expected Outcomes of Medical Nutrition Therapy

Clinical Outcome Assessment Factors	Expected Outcome of Therapy	Ideal/Goal Value Renal Insufficiency	Ideal/Goal Value Dialysis	Ideal/Goal Value Transplant
• Biochemical Parameters —BUN (mg/dL) —Albumin (g/dL) —Potassium (mEq/L) —Phosphorus (mg/dL) —Calcium (mg/dL) —Cholesterol (mg/dL) —Serum glucose (mg/dL) (premeal)	—Biochemical parameters stabilized at or progressing toward goal values	—BUN < 60 —Albumin ≥ 3.5 —Potassium 3.5–5.5 —Phosphorus 2.5–6.0 —Calcium 8.5–10.5 —Cholesterol 150–300 —Glucose 60–105	—BUN < 50 —Albumin ≥ 3.5 —Potassium 3.5–5.5 —Phosphorus 4.5–6.0 —Calcium 8.5–10.5 —Cholesterol 150–300 —Glucose 60–105	—BUN 7.2–10.2 —Albumin ≥ 3.5 —Potassium 3.5–5.5 —Phosphorus 2.5–6.0 —Calcium 8.5–10.5 —Cholesterol 150–300 —Glucose 60–105
• Hematological Parameters —Hematocrit (%) —Hemoglobin (g/dL)	—Adequate erythropoiesis maintained	—Hematocrit > 30 —Hemoglobin 10–14	—Hematocrit > 30 —Hemoglobin 10–14	—Hematocrit 32–42 —Hemoglobin 10–14
• Anthropometrics —Dry weight gains —Interdialytic fluid gains (hemodialysis) • Clinical Signs and Symptoms	—Dry weight increasing as appropriate (see Recommended Weight Gain for Pregnant Women table) —Fluid gains achieved/ maintained at goal —Maternal muscle and fat stores maintained —Level of functional ability maintained —Good appetite maintained —Appropriate blood pressure control maintained	—Based on initial BMI and pregnancy trimester (see Recommended Weight Gain for Pregnant Women table) —Not Applicable —Adequate muscle/fat stores —Optimum functional ability —Minimum GI symptoms —Food intake > 80% recommended needs —Blood pressure within appropriate limits	—Based on initial BMI and pregnancy trimester (see Recommended Weight Gain for Pregnant Women table) —Fluid gains 1–2 kg (hemodialysis) —Adequate muscle/fat stores —Optimum functional ability —Minimum GI symptoms —Food intake > 80% recommended needs —Blood pressure within appropriate limits	—Based on initial BMI and pregnancy trimester (see Recommended Weight Gain for Pregnant Women table) —Not Applicable —Adequate muscle/fat stores —Optimum functional ability —Minimum GI symptoms —Food intake > 80% recommended needs —Blood pressure within appropriate limits
Patient/Caregiver Behavioral Outcomes • Food selection/meal planning • Nutrient needs • Weight gain • Potential food/drug interactions • Exercise	—Exhibits positive changes in food selection and amounts —If diabetic, times meals and snacks appropriately —Identifies foods high in calories, protein, sodium, potassium, phosphorus, iron, and folate content as indicated —Maintains appropriate fluid intake —Verbalizes appropriate weight gain during pregnancy —Verbalizes potential food/drug interactions —If no medical limitations, gradually increases or continues physical activity level	**MNT Goals** 1. Makes appropriate food choices and takes medications as prescribed 2. Maintains appropriate protein intake 3. Maintains lab values within acceptable limits 4. If diabetic, maintains stable glucose levels through appropriate dietary practices 5. Maintains appropriate weight gain pattern 6. If no medical limitations, maintenance of an exercise program	**MNT Goals** 1. Makes appropriate food choices and takes medications as prescribed 2. Maintains adequate protein intake 3. Maintains lab values within acceptable limits 4. If diabetic, maintains stable glucose levels through appropriate dietary practices 5. Maintains appropriate weight gain pattern 6. If no medical limitations, maintenance of an exercise program	**MNT Goals** 1. Makes appropriate food choices and takes medications as prescribed 2. Maintains appropriate intake of calories and protein 3. Maintains lab values within acceptable limits 4. If diabetic, maintains stable glucose levels through appropriate dietary practices 5. Maintains appropriate weight gain pattern 6. If no medical limitations, maintenance of an exercise program

Minimum Baseline Data Needed for Medical Nutrition Therapy

Factor	Data Needed
Laboratory Values with Dates (within 30 days of session)	1. BUN, creatinine 2. Albumin 3. Sodium, potassium, phosphorus, calcium 4. Serum glucose 5. Serum bicarbonate 6. PTH, if available 7. Hematocrit/hemoglobin 8. Ferritin, transferrin saturation, serum iron 9. Dialysis adequacy and PET results, if appropriate 10. Urinalysis results as appropriate (e.g., volume, urea, protein, sodium) 11. Creatinine clearance or GFR 12. Others as appropriate (e.g., lipid profile, glycosylated hemoglobin, vitamin B12, folate)
Health Care Team's Goals for Patient	1. Patient prognosis 2. Prognosis for pregnancy 3. Expected outcome of nutrition therapy
Medical History	1. Disease/condition causing renal failure 2. History of renal disease and treatment 3. Date of conception 4. History of prior pregnancies and outcomes/complications 5. Concurrent medical conditions (e.g., diabetes, HIV, cardiovascular disease, GI problems, hypertension, hyperlipidemia) 6. Any other medical or physical conditions with potential nutritional implications (e.g., surgery, infection, CVA, blindness, neuropathies)
Medications/Therapies	1. Current treatment mode for ESRD 2. Type of dialysis therapy and prescription if appropriate 3. Diet order, tube-feeding order, parenteral nutrition order, and/or IDPN/IPN order 4. Any other treatments or therapies that may affect nutritional intake or status 5. Immunosuppressants 6. Antihypertensives, diuretics 7. Anticoagulants 8. Phosphate binders 9. Vitamin/mineral supplements 10. Any other medications with food/drug interactions or nutritional impact (e.g., diabetes medications, GI medications, steroids)
Psychosocial Issues	1. Learning disabilities 2. Vision, hearing abilities 3. Cultural or language barriers 4. Mental status
Guidelines for Exercise	1. Medical clearance for exercise 2. Exercise limitations, if any

Initial Nutrition Assessment

Session: *Initial*　　　　　Length: *60–90 minutes*　　　Time: *Within 1 month of diagnosis of pregnancy*

Factor	Assessments
Clinical Data	1. Review Minimum Baseline Data. 2. Obtain current height, pregravida dry weight, and BMI. 3. Obtain weight history, recent weight changes, and weight goals. 4. Determine pregravida IBW and/or UBW adjusted for amputation or obesity, and percentage IBW and/or percentage UBW (see Appendix B). 5. Determine appropriate weight gain pattern per BMI (see Recommended Weight Gain for Pregnant Women table). 6. Assess muscle and fat stores, presence of edema. 7. Assess for physical signs of nutrient deficiencies/excesses or increased needs (e.g., decubiti, poor wound healing, thinning hair, pale conjunctiva, cheilosis). 8. Determine nitrogen balance using urea kinetics, if appropriate (see Appendix D). 9. Assess blood pressure control.
Dietary Evaluation	1. Determine previous dietary instruction and practices. 2. Determine usual food intake and pattern of intake. 3. Assess appetite, GI issues, tolerance of oral intake, and food allergies/intolerances. 4. Assess feeding issues (e.g., chewing, swallowing). 5. Determine use of vitamin/mineral, herbal, or other nutrition supplements. 6. Determine alcohol/drug/tobacco use and history. 7. For PD, determine glucose absorption and calories from dialysate (see Appendix C). 8. Assess intake of calories, protein, sodium, potassium, phosphorus, calcium, fluids, and other nutrients as indicated (e.g., caffeine). 9. Assess diet order, tube-feeding order, parenteral nutrition order, and/or IDPN/IPN order for appropriateness.
Functional Ability/Exercise	1. Determine level of functional ability and recent changes. 2. Assess ability to feed self and needs for assistance. 3. Determine activity level and exercise habits. 4. Determine physical or motivational limitations to exercise.
Psychosocial and Economic Issues	1. Assess living situation, cooking facilities, finances, educational background, employment, literacy, and any other factors that may affect availability of food. 2. Assess ethnic or religious belief considerations. 3. Assess availability of support systems. 4. Determine whether other relevant psychosocial or economic issues exist.
Knowledge, Skill Level, Attitudes, and Motivation	1. Assess basic knowledge level of dietary guidelines for patient's mode of treatment. 2. Assess basic knowledge level of nutritional needs in pregnancy. 3. Assess attitudes toward nutrition and health. 4. Determine patient's willingness and ability to learn and make appropriate changes.

Initial Nutrition Intervention: Renal Insufficiency

Session: *Initial*   Length: *60–90 minutes*   Time: *Within 1 month of diagnosis of pregnancy*

Factor	Interventions
Management Goals	1. Identify management goals of health care team. 2. Identify patient goals and expectations.
Nutrition Prescription	1. Calories—individualized to maintain appropriate weight gain; use basal energy expenditure $\times$ activity factor (1.2–1.4) or > 35 kcal/kg pregravida IBW (include an additional 300 calories per day for second and third trimesters). 2. Protein—based on creatinine clearance, GFR, urinary protein losses (0.6–1.0 g/kg pregravida IBW + 10 gm); to maintain BUN < 60, albumin $\geq$ 3.5 (50% from high biological value animal and/or plant sources). 4. Sodium—individualized, or 1–3 g/day. 5. Potassium—individualized per lab values. 6. Phosphorus—individualized per lab values, appx. 800–1200 mg/day; may require phosphate binder therapy. 7. Calcium—individualized per calcium, phosphorus, and PTH lab values; appx. 1200 mg/day 8. Fluids—as desired to maintain appropriate hydration status. 9. Vitamin/mineral supplementation (See Vitamin and Mineral Recommendations table.)
Self-Management Skills	1. Discuss simple definitions and examples of calories, protein, sodium, and other nutrients as appropriate (e.g., carbohydrates, fats, potassium, phosphorus, calcium, iron, folate, fluids). 2. Discuss basic dietary guidelines for renal insufficiency. 3. For diabetes, discuss basic dietary guidelines and timing of meals and snacks, if indicated. 4. Discuss appropriate weight gain pattern during pregnancy. 5. Discuss laboratory tests and significance of results. 6. Discuss use and effect of vitamin supplements. 7. Discuss food/drug interactions as indicated. 8. Discuss dangers associated with the use of alcohol and other harmful substances in pregnancy. 9. Discuss role and effect of diet and medications in renal disease and pregnancy. 10. Discuss importance of maternal nutrition, blood pressure control, and blood glucose regulation on pregnancy outcome. 11. Discuss dietary modifications that may help relieve nausea, vomiting, heartburn, constipation, and other GI symptoms. 12. Assess comprehension of education provided and projected compliance.
Functional Ability/Exercise	1. Provide necessary referrals for assistance with self-feeding and other activities of daily living (e.g., OT, PT, speech therapy). 2. Discuss exercise recommendations, if appropriate.
Behavioral Goals	1. Address eating and exercise behaviors. 2. Identify and summarize short-term behavioral goals that are specific and achievable. 3. Establish follow-up plan.
Communication	1. Document current nutritional status, plan of care, and goals of MNT. 2. Report recommendations/concerns to appropriate health care team member (e.g., MD, RN, pharmacist, social worker). 3. Provide information regarding nutrition prescription and dietary guidelines to referral source, extended-care facility, home health care agencies, if appropriate.

Initial Nutrition Intervention: Dialysis

Session: *Initial*   Length: *60–90 minutes*   Time: *Within 1 month of diagnosis of pregnancy*

Factor	Interventions
Management Goals	1. Identify management goals of health care team. 2. Identify patient goals and expectations.
Nutrition Prescription	1. Calories—individualized to maintain appropriate weight gain; use basal energy expenditure × activity factor (1.2–1.4) or 30–35 kcal/kg pregravida IBW (include an additional 300 calories per day for second and third trimesters). 2. Protein = 1.1–1.4 g/kg pregravida IBW +10 gm (hemodialysis); 1.2–1.5 g/kg pregravida IBW + 10 gm (peritoneal dialysis); may be higher depending on stress or metabolic needs. 3. Sodium—individualized, appx. 2–3 g/day (hemodialysis); 2–4 g/day (peritoneal dialysis) 4. Potassium—individualized, appx. 40 mg/kg pregravida IBW (hemodialysis); restricted only by lab values (peritoneal dialysis). 5. Phosphorus—individualized per lab values, appx.1200 mg/day; may require phosphate binder therapy. 6. Calcium—individualized per calcium, phosphorus, and PTH lab values; appx. 1000–1200 mg/day; dependent on dialysate calcium concentration and phosphate binder use. 7. Fluids—1000–2000 mL + urine output per interdialytic interval to maintain 1–2 kg interdialytic weight gain (hemodialysis); to maintain fluid balance (peritoneal dialysis). 8. Vitamin/mineral supplementation (see Vitamin and Mineral Recommendations table)
Self-Management Skills	1. Discuss simple definitions and examples of calories, protein, and other nutrients as appropriate (e.g., sodium, potassium, phosphorus, calcium, iron, folate, fluids). 2. Discuss basic dietary guidelines for ESRD. 3. For diabetes, discuss basic dietary guidelines and timing of meals and snacks, if indicated. 4. Discuss appropriate dry weight gain pattern during pregnancy. 5. For hemodialysis, discuss appropriate level of interdialytic fluid gains. 6. Discuss laboratory tests and significance of results. 7. Discuss use and effect of phosphate binders. 8. Discuss use and effect of vitamin supplements. 9. Discuss food/drug interactions as indicated. 10. Discuss dangers associated with the use of alcohol and other harmful substances in pregnancy. 11. Discuss role and effect of diet, medications, and dialysis in renal disease and pregnancy. 12. Discuss importance of maternal nutrition, blood pressure control, and blood glucose regulation on pregnancy outcome. 13. Discuss dietary modifications that may help relieve nausea, vomiting, heartburn, constipation, and other GI symptoms. 14. Assess comprehension of education provided and projected compliance.
Functional Ability/Exercise	1. Provide necessary referrals for assistance with self-feeding and other activities of daily living (e.g OT, PT, speech therapy). 2. Discuss exercise recommendations, if appropriate.
Behavioral Goals	1. Address eating and exercise behaviors. 2. Identify and summarize short-term behavioral goals that are specific and achievable. 3. Establish follow-up plan.
Communication	1. Document current nutritional status, plan of care, and goals of MNT. 2. Report recommendations/concerns to appropriate health care team member (e.g., MD, RN, pharmacist, social worker). 3. Provide information regarding nutrition prescription and dietary guidelines to extended-care facility, home health care facilities, if appropriate.

Initial Nutrition Intervention: Transplantation

Session: *Initial*   Length: *60–90 minutes*   Time: *Within 1 month of diagnosis of pregnancy*

Factor	Interventions
Management Goals	1. Identify management goals of health care team. 2. Identify patient goals and expectations.
Nutrition Prescription	1. Calories—individualized to maintain appropriate weight gain; use basal energy expenditure $\times$ activity factor (1.2 to 1.4) or 25–35 kcal/kg pregravida IBW (include an additional 300 calories per day for second and third trimesters). 2. Protein = 1.0–1.2 g/kg pregravida IBW + 10 gm; may be higher depending on stress or metabolic needs 3. Carbohydrate—50–60% total calories; limit concentrated sweets and emphasize complex carbohydrates 6. Sodium—individualized; appx. 2–4 g/day 7. Potassium—restrict to 2–4 g/day if hyperkalemic 8. Phosphorus—1200 mg/day 9. Calcium—1200–1500 mg/day 10. Fluids—as desired 11. Vitamin/mineral supplementation (see Vitamin and Mineral Recommendations table)
Self-Management Skills	1. Discuss simple definitions and examples of calories, protein, and other nutrients as appropriate (e.g., carbohydrates, sodium, potassium, phosphorus, calcium, iron, folate). 2. Discuss basic dietary guidelines for pregnancy. 3. For diabetes, discuss basic dietary guidelines and timing of meals and snacks, if indicated. 4. Discuss appropriate weight gain pattern during pregnancy. 5. Discuss laboratory tests and significance of results. 6. Discuss use and effect of vitamin supplements. 7. Discuss food/drug interactions as indicated. 8. Discuss dangers associated with the use of alcohol and other harmful substances in pregnancy. 9. Discuss role and effect of diet and medications in renal disease and pregnancy. 10. Discuss importance of maternal nutrition, blood pressure control, and blood glucose regulation on pregnancy outcome. 11. Discuss dietary modifications that may help relieve nausea, vomiting, heartburn, constipation, and other GI symptoms. 12. Assess comprehension of education provided and projected compliance.
Functional Ability/Exercise	1. Provide necessary referrals for assistance with self-feeding and other activities of daily living (e.g., OT, PT, speech therapy). 2. Discuss exercise recommendations, if appropriate.
Behavioral Goals	1. Address eating and exercise behaviors. 2. Identify and summarize short-term behavioral goals that are specific and achievable. 3. Establish follow-up plan.
Communication	1. Document current nutritional status, plan of care, and goals of MNT. 2. Report recommendations/concerns to appropriate health care team member (e.g., MD, RN, pharmacist, social worker). 3. Provide information regarding nutrition prescription and dietary guidelines to extended-care facility, home health care facilities, if appropriate.

Follow-up Nutrition Assessment: All Treatment Modalities

Session: *Follow-up Sessions*   Length: *30–45 minutes*   Time: *Weekly for dialysis, monthly for transplants and renal insufficiency*

Factor	Assessments
Clinical Data	1. Review changes in medical status and recent/planned therapies (e.g., medication, dialysis, surgery). 2. Review any new or updated laboratory data. 3. Assess changes in weight. For dialysis, assess changes in dry weight and interdialytic weight changes, if appropriate. 4. Assess muscle and fat stores, presence of edema. 5. Assess for physical signs of nutrient deficiencies/excesses or increased needs (e.g., decubiti, poor wound healing, thinning hair, pale conjunctiva, cheilosis). 6. Review dialysis adequacy and PET results, if appropriate. 7. Assess blood pressure control. 8. Assess effectiveness of previous nutrition intervention.
Dietary Evaluation	1. Determine current GI or feeding issues or concerns. 2. Assess changes in patient's food intake and/or appetite. 3. For PD, determine glucose absorption and calories from dialysate (see Appendix C). 4. Assess dietary intake and/or nutritional support intake for adequacy and appropriateness.
Functional Ability/Exercise	1. Assess changes in functional ability. 2. Assess changes in activity level or exercise habits.
Behavioral Outcomes	1. Assess understanding of simple definitions and examples of calories, protein, and other nutrients as appropriate (e.g., carbohydrates, sodium, potassium, phosphorus, calcium, fluids). 2. Assess understanding of basic dietary guidelines discussed. 3. For diabetes, assess understanding of basic dietary guidelines and timing of meals and snacks. 4. Assess understanding of appropriate weight gain pattern during pregnancy. 5. For hemodialysis, assess understanding of appropriate level of interdialytic fluid gains. 6. Assess understanding of laboratory tests and significance of results. 7. Assess understanding of use and effect of phosphate binders, if appropriate. 8. Assess understanding of use and effect of vitamin supplements. 9. Assess understanding of food/drug interactions as indicated. 10. Assess understanding of dangers associated with the use of alcohol and other harmful substances in pregnancy. 11. Assess understanding of role and effect of diet, medications, and therapy mode on renal disease and pregnancy. 12. Assess understanding of importance of maternal nutrition, blood pressure control, and blood glucose regulation on pregnancy outcome. 13. Assess understanding of dietary modifications that may help relieve nausea, vomiting, heartburn, constipation, and other GI symptoms. 14. Determine further improvements that can be made in the quality of the diet.
Behavioral Goals	1. Assess achievement of prior behavioral goals. 2. Determine willingness and ability to make further changes.

Follow-up Nutrition Intervention: All Treatment Modalities

Session: *Follow-up* Length: *30–45 minutes* Time: *Weekly for dialysis, monthly for transplants and renal insufficiency*

Factor	Interventions
Nutrition Prescription	1. Provide feedback on laboratory results, blood pressure control, changes in weight. 2. Provide feedback on food/meal plan, food choices, and portions. 3. Recommend changes in nutrient intake or habits that can improve outcomes. 4. Adjust MNT, as appropriate.
Self-Management Skills	1. Review and reinforce self-management skills from prior session. 2. Provide and review educational materials as appropriate. 3. If medications change, discuss potential food/drug interaction and impact on pregnancy. 4. Assess comprehension of education provided and projected compliance.
Functional Ability/Exercise	1. Refer to OT, PT, speech therapy as appropriate. 2. Discuss changes in exercise recommendations, if appropriate.
Behavioral Goals	1. Reset short-term behavioral goals that are specific and achievable. 2. Review and reinforce long-term goals. 3. Establish follow-up plan.
Communication	1. Document current nutritional status, plan of care, and goals of MNT. 2. Report recommendations/concerns to appropriate health care team member (e.g., MD, RN, pharmacist, social worker). 3. Provide information regarding nutrition prescription and dietary guidelines to extended-care facility, home health care facilities, if appropriate.

Recommended Weight Gain for Pregnant Women Based on Body Mass Index (BMI)*

Weight Category Based on BMI	Total Weight Gain		1st Trimester Gain			2nd and 3rd Trimester Weekly Gain	
	lbs	kg	lbs	kg		lbs	kg
Underweight: BMI < 19.8	28–40	12.5–18	5	2.3		1. 07	0.49
Normal weight: BMI 19.8–26.0	25–35	11.5–16	3.5	1. 6		0.97	0.44
Overweight: BMI 26.0–29.0	15–25	7–11.5	2	0.9		0.67	0.30
Obese: BMI > 29.0	at least 15	6	NA[†]	NA		0.50	0.23

Adapted from Nutrition During Pregnancy: ACOG Technical Bulletin Number 179-April 1993. *IntJGynedolObstet* 43:67–74,1993.

* BMI =weight (kg)/height (m)^2

[†] NA = Not Available

Vitamin and Mineral Recommendations

Nutrient	Standards for Normal Pregnancy Suggested Standard for Renal Insufficienty and Transplantation	Suggested Standards for Pregnancy in Hemodialysis	Potential Effects on Pregnancy
Vitamins			
A (μg)	800	No supplement	Excess: Spontaneous abortion, birth defects involving the fetal bone, urinary tract, and CNS, maternal liver damage Def: Possible eye abnormalities and impaired vision
D (μg)	10	$1,25(OH)_2D_3$ if low serum levels	Excess: Hypercalcemia in infant which can lead to neonatal seizures Def: disorders of calcium metablism in newborn, reduction in bone calcification or bone density, neonatal hypocalcemia and tetany, tooth enamel hypoplasia, maternal osteomalacia
E (mg)	8	No supplement	Excess: Spontaneous abortion
C (mg)	70	$\geq$ 170	Excess: Metabolic dependency in offspring can lead to neonatal scurvy Def: Premature birth, low birth weight
Thiamine (mg)	1.5	3.0	Def: Congenital beriberi if deficiency severe
Riboflavin (mg)	1.6	3.4	Unknown
Niacin (mg)	17	Unknown, $\geq$ 20	Unknown
B6 (mg)	2.2	Unknown, $\geq$ 5	Def: Unsatisfactory Apgar scores, maternal depression
B12 (mg)	2.2	NA	Def: Prematurity, CNS abnormalities, maternal megaloblastic anemia
Biotin (μg)	30–100*	600	Unknown
Folic Acid (mg)	0.4	1. 8	Def: Neural tube defect, low birth weight or small for gestational age infants, maternal megaloblastic anemia
Minerals			
Calcium (mg)	1200	From Phosphate binder, monitor Calcium levels	Def: Depletion of maternal skeleton, increased risk of maternal hypertension and pregnancy-induced toxemia
Phosphorus (mg)	1200	1200 from diet	Unknown
Magnesium (mg)	300	Unknown, 200–300	Unknown
Iron (mg)	30	200 or per Iron studies	Def: Preterm delivery, low birth weight, reduced fetal iron storage with increased risk of anemia in infancy, maternal iron-defieiency anemia
Zinc (mg)	15	15	Def: Preterm delivery, low birth weight or small for gestational age infants, increased risk of fetal malformations, prolonged labor, increased risk for pregnancy-induced hypertension
Carnitine (mg)	NA	Unknown, 330	Unknown

* Estimated Safe and Adequate Daily Dietary Intake

Bibliography

Abrams B. Weight gain and energy intake during pregnancy. *Clin Obstet Gynecol.* 1994;37(3): 515–527.

American Diabetes Association Position Statement: Screening for Diabetes. *DiabetesCare.* 1997; 20(Suppl 1):S22–S23.

American Diabetes Association. *Maximizing the Role of Nutrition in Diabetes Management.* Alexandria, Va: American Diabetes Association, Inc;1994.

Barri YM, Al-Furayn O, Qunibi WY, Rahman F. Pregnancy in women on regular hemodialysis. *Dial&Transplant.* 1991;20(11):652–656,695.

Bobak IM, Lowdermilk DL, Jensen MD, eds. *Maternity Nursing.* 4th ed. St. Louis, Mo: Mosby, 1995.

Brookhyser J, Kinzner C, Pahre S. A case study of two successful pregnancies in a patient with end-stage renal disease. *JRenalNutr.* 1996;6(1):26–33.

Brookhyser J, Wiggins K. Medical nutrition therapy in pregnancy and kidney disease. *AdvRenalReplaceTher.* 1998;5(1):53–63.

Brown ML, ed. *Present Knowledge in Nutrition.* 6th ed. Washington, DC: International Life Sciences Institute;1990.

The Chicago Dietetic Association, The South Suburban Dietetic Association, and Dietitians of Canada. *Manual of Clinical Dietetics.* 6th ed. Chicago, Ill: American Dietetic Association; 2000.

Cunningham FG, Cox SM, Harstad TW, Mason RA, Pritchard JA. Chronic renal disease and pregnancy outcome. *AmJObstetGynecol.* 1990;163(2):453–459.

Davison JM. Dialysis, transplantation, and pregnancy. *AmJKidneyDis.* 1991;17(2):127–132.

Davison JM. Pregnancy in renal allograft recipients: Problems, prognosis and practicalities. *Bailliere'sClinObstetGynaecol.* 1994;8(2):501–525.

Dunbeck D, Klopstein K, Heroux J, Brencick K. Peritoneal dialysis patient completes successful pregnancy. *ANNAJ.* 1992;19(3):269,272.

Elliott JP, O'Keeffe DF, Schon DA, Cherem LB. Dialysis in pregnancy: A critical review. *ObstetGynecolSurvey.* 1991;46(6):319–324.

Farkas-Hirsch R, ed. *Intensive Diabetes Management.* Alexandria, Va: American Diabetes Association;1995.

Grossman SD, Hou S, Moretti M, Saran M. Nutrition in the pregnant dialysis patient. *JRenalNutr.* 1993;3(2):56–66.

Hayslett JP, Reece EA. Managing diabetic patients with nephropathy and other vascular complications. *Bailliere'sClinObstetGynaecol.* 1994;8(2):405–424.

Henderson N. Nutritional management of pregnancy in a chronic hemodialysis patient with insulin-dependent diabetes mellitus. *JRenalNutr.* 1996;6(4):222–228.

Holley JL, Bernardini J, Quadri KHM, Greenberg A, Laifer SA. Pregnancy outcomes in a prospective matched control study of pregnancy and renal disease. *ClinNephrol.* 1996;45(2):77–82.

Hou SH. Pregnancy in chronic renal insufficiency and end-stage renal disease. *AmJKidneyDis.* 1999;33(2):235–252.

Hou SH. Pregnancy in women on haemodialysis and peritoneal dialysis. *Bailliere's ClinObsteGynaecol.* 1994;8(2):481–500.

Hou S, Grossman S. Pregnancy in chronic dialysis patients. *SeminDial.* 1990;3:224–229.

Hou S, Orlowski J, Pahl M, Ambrose S, Hussey M, Wong D. Pregnancy in women with end-stage renal disease: Treatment of anemia and premature labor. *AmJKidneyDis.* 1993;21(1):16–22.

Imbasciati E, Ponticelli C. Pregnancy and renal disease: Predictors for fetal and maternal outcome. *AmJNephrol.* 1991;11:353–362.

Kopple JD, Massry SG, eds. *Nutritional Management of Renal Disease.* Baltimore, Md: Williams & Wilkins;1997.

Lebovitz HE, ed. *Therapy for Diabetes Mellitus and Related Disorders.* 2nd ed. Alexandria, Va: American Diabetes Association, Inc; 1994.

Levine DZ, ed. *Care of the Renal Patient.* 2nd ed. Philadelphia, Pa: WB Saunders Company; 1991.

Lindheimer MD, Katz AI. Gestation in women with kidney disease: Prognosis and management. *Bailliere'sClinObstetGynaecol.* 1994;8(2):387–404.

Mahan LK, Escott-Stump S. *Krause's Food, Nutrition and Diet Therapy.* 9th ed. Philadelphia, Pa: WB Saunders;1996.

Maurer G, Abriloa D. Pregnancy following renal transplant. *JPerinatNeonatalNurs.* 1994;8(1): 28–36.

McCann L, Yates L, Ezaki-Yamaguchi J, Akiyama P. Forms to monitor and assess nutritional status of renal patients. *JRenalNutr.* 1995;5(3):151–155.

McCann L. *Subjective Global Assessment.* Redwood City, Calif: Satellite Dialysis Centers, Inc;1997.

McCann L. Subjective global assessment as it pertains to the nutritional status of dialysis patients. *Dial&Transplant.* 1996;25(4):190–199, 202, 225.

Nutrition during pregnancy: ACOG technical bulletin number 179—April 1993. *IntJGynecolObstet.* 1993;43:67–74.

Perry LA. A multidisciplinary approach to the management of pregnant patients with end-stage renal disease. *JPerinatNeonatalNurs.* 1994;8(1):12–19.

Smolin LA, Grosvenor MB. *Nutrition: Science and Applications.* 2nd ed. Orlando, Fla: Saunders College Publishing;1997.

Stover J, ed. *A Clinical Guide to Nutrition Care in End-Stage Renal Disease.* 2nd ed. Chicago, Ill: The American Dietetic Association;1994.

Vidal ML, Ursu M, Martinez A, Roland SS, Wibmer E, Pereira D, Subiza K, Alonso W, Seijas L, Piazze S, Lisorio L, Falconi JP, Canessa R, Laborda L, Dibello N. Nutritional control of pregnant women on chronic hemodiaysis. *JRenalNutr.* 1998;8(3):150–156.

Wada L, King JC. Trace element nutrition during pregnancy. *ClinObsteGynecol.* 1994;37(3): 574–586.

Worthington-Roberts B, Wiliams SR. *Nutrition in Pregnancy and Lactation.* 4th ed. St. Louis. Mo:Times Mirror/Mosby College Publishing;1989.

Appendixes

Appendix A
Abbreviations

ABW	adjusted body weight
appx	approximately
BMI	body mass index
BSA	body surface area
BUN	blood urea nitrogen
BW	body weight
CAPD	continuous ambulatory peritoneal dialysis
CAVH	continuous arteriovenous hemodialysis
CHD	coronary heart disease
CO_2	carbon dioxide
CVA	cerebrovascular accident
DOQI	Dialysis Outcomes Quality Initiative
EPO	erythropoietin
ESRD	end-stage renal disease
F	female
GER	glomerular filtration rate
GI	gastrointestinal
HDL	high density lipoprotein
HgbA1C	hemoglobin Al C (glycosylated hemoglobin)
HIV	human immunodeficiency virus
ht	height
LBW	ideal body weight
IDL	intermediate density lipoprotein
IDPN	intradialytic parenteral nutrition
IPN	intrperitoneal nutrition

IV	intravenous
Kcal	kilocalories
kg	kilograms
Kt/V	measure of dose of dialysis
LDL	low density lipoprotein
M	male
MD	medical doctor
MINT	medical nutrition therapy
MUFA	monounsaturated fatty acids
NCEP	National Cholesterol Education Program
NHLBI	National Heart, Lung, and Blood Institute
NIH	National Institutes of Health
NKF	National Kidney Foundation
nPCR	normalized protein catabolic rate
nPNA	normalized protein equivalent of nitrogen appearance
OT	occupational therapist
PCR	protein catabolic rate
PET	peritoneal equilibration test
PNA	protein equivalent of nitrogen appearance
PT	physical therapist
PTH	parathyroid hormone
PUPA	polyunsaturated fatty acidss
RN	registered nurse
RPG	Renal Practice Group
SGOT	serum glutamic oxaloacetic transaminase

SGPT	serum glutamic pyruvic transaminase	URR	urea reduction ratio
TPN	total parenteral nutrition	US RDA	United States recommended daily allowance
UBW	usual body weight	VLDL	very low density lipoprotein
UNA	urea nitrogen appearance	wt	weight

Appendix B
Adjustment in Body Weight

Obesity

Caloric and protein requirements are typically determined with formulas that use an individual's current body weight. For energy requirements, the Harris-Benedict equations are frequently employed and provide an estimate of the resting energy expenditure (REE) for the individual. In a person whose weight is well above desirable weight, however, there is no consensus regarding the most appropriate way to determine energy needs.

In obesity, it has been common practice to adjust body weight in reference to ideal body weight (IBW) or desirable weight, and then apply the Harris-Benedict equations, rather than use the actual (obese) weight. The rationale behind this method is that using actual (obese) body weight will overestimate REE because an obese person has a greater percentage of body fat (compared to a person at desirable weight), and body fat is much less metabolically active and requires fewer calories.[1,2] On the other hand, using desirable body weight to calculate REE in obese persons will underestimate required calories.

It has been found that FFM correlates closely with REE in normal weight and obese subjects,[2-10] and thus the common practice has been to consider the increase in FFM that accompanies accrual of obese tissue and adjust the desirable body weight accordingly. Various studies have looked at the percentage of FFM in obese tissue and estimates range from 22–33% FFM for women and 19–38% FFM for men. To adjust body weight in obese subjects using this rationale, the following formula can be employed:[2,3,4,10]

Formula 1: Adjusted Weight (kg) = [(ABW − IBW) × FFM factor] + IBW

Where:

> ABW = actual body weight
> IBW = ideal body weight/desirable body weight
> FFM factor = 0.22–0.33 Women
>   0.19–0.38 Men

This method of adjustment is based only on theory. There are no studies that validate the methodology in the literature.

Several researchers have looked at REE in populations including obese subjects and have developed alternate formulas to the Harris-Benedict equations.[1,7,8,11,12] Reviews of several of these formulas have shown that the Harris-Benedict equations are as predictive of REE for the populations studied (which included obese subjects) as other commonly used methods.[10,13] Recent review of the data from the Harris-Benedict study has shown that using the Harris-Benedict equations with actual body weight is most likely valid in the moderately obese, up to a BMI of 30–35.[14] For individuals with BMIs of more than 35–40, the Harris-Benedict equations appear to overestimate REE by approximately 15% when actual body weight is used.[15]

Determination of protein requirements in obesity has not been addressed in the literature except in the issue of weight loss using very low calorie diets. There is no data regarding the best methodology for calculating maintenance protein needs in the obese individual. The rationale for adjusting body weight for protein is similar to that for adjusting for caloric needs. As body weight increases, protein-containing tissues will increase and an individual's protein requirements could be expected to increase as well. The degree to which protein needs increase is not known. It may be proportional to the increase in FFM, but there is no data to support this.

There is currently no validated method for calculating energy and protein needs in the obese individual. Each person's nutrient needs must be assessed individually. In some situations, it may appear to be most appropriate to adjust body weight for FFM before determining caloric or protein needs. In other situations, using actual body weight or IBW may seem more appropriate. The practitioner must use his or her own judgment and expertise in determining the most appropriate method to use in assessing a particular individual's needs.

Amputations

Before one can calculate caloric and protein requirements for patients with amputations, ideal body weight also needs to be adjusted. Table B.1 lists the percentage of total body weight contributed by certain segments of the body.[16]

Table B.1

Body Segment	Average Percentage (%) of Total Body Weight
Entire arm	5.0
Upper arm (to elbow)	2.7
Forearm	1.6
Hand	0.7
Entire leg	16.0
Thigh	10.1
Calf	4.4
Foot	1.5

If several segments are included in the amputation, such as the lower leg consisting of calf and foot, then the percentages are summed to equal the total percentage of the amputation. For example, with a lower leg amputation, the percentages for calf and foot segments would be summed to yield a total amputation weight percentage of 5.9%.

Calculating Ideal Body Weight

Limb weight must be taken into account in the determination of ideal body weight (IBW). In estimating the ideal weight range for a patient with an amputation, find the IBW range for the patient's height, multiply it by [100 − (%weight of amputation)], then divide the result by 100.

Calculating BMI

BMI can be calculated by first calculating an **estimate of the full body weight** including the missing limb segments using the following formula:

Formula 2: Estimated BW(kg) $= \dfrac{\text{measured weight}}{[100 - (\% \text{ weight of amputation})]} \times 100$

The **adjusted BMI** can then be calculated by substituting the estimated body weight in the equation for BMI.

Formula 3: $\mathrm{BMI_{adj}} = \dfrac{\text{Estimated BW}}{\mathrm{Ht}^2}$

Where:

   height (Ht) is measured in meters.

   By substituting Formula 2 into Formula 3 for Estimated BW, the following formula is derived for calculating **adjusted BMI** ($\mathrm{BMI_{adj}}$) directly:

Formula 4: $\mathrm{BMI_{adj}} = \dfrac{\text{measured weight}}{\mathrm{Ht}^2 \times [100 - (\%\ \text{weight of amputation})]} \times 100$

Adjusting Volume[17]

1. An estimate of full body weight is first determined using Formula 2.
2. This weight is then used in the appropriate formula for calculating volume to obtain the estimated volume including the missing limb segments, or the **estimated full body volume**. See Appendix D for volume formulas.
3. Divide the full body volume by the full body weight. This yields the proportion of water in 1 kilogram of the patient's weight (number of liters/kg). It is assumed that the proportion of water is the same throughout the entire body.
4. Multiply this proportion times the actual postamputation weight to determine the **volume adjusted for amputation**.

References

1. Owen OE, Kavle E, Owen RS, et al. A reappraisal of caloric requirements in healthy women. *AmJClinNutr.* 1986;44:1–19.

2. Forbes GB, Welle SL. Lean body mass in obesity. *IntJObes.* 1983;7:99–107.

3. Webster JD, Hesp R, Garrow JS. The composition of excess weight in obese women estimated by bodydensity, total body water and total body potassium. *HumNutr.* 1984;38C:299–306.

4. James WPT, Bailes J, Davies HL, Dauncey MJ. Elevated metabolic rates in obesity. *Lancet.* 1978;1:1122–1125.

5. Bernstein RS, Thornton JC, Yang MU, et al. Prediction of the resting metabolic rate in obese patients. *AmJClinNutr.* 1983;37:595–602.

6. Ravussin E, Burnand B, Schutz Y, Jequier E. Twenty-four-hour energy expenditure and resting metabolicr ate in obese, moderately obese, and control subjects. *AmJClinNutr.* 1982;35:566–573.

7. Cunningham JJ. Body composition as a determinant of energy expenditure: A synthetic review and a proposed general prediction equation. *AmJClinNutr.* 1991;54:963–969.

8. Mifflin MD, St Jeor ST, Hill LA, Scott BJ, Daugherty SA, Koh YO. A new predictive equation for resting energy expenditure in healthy individuals. *AmJClinNutr.* 1990;51:241–247.

9. Fredrix EW, Soeters PB, Deerenberg IM, Kester AD, von Meyenfeldt MF, Saris WH. Resting and sleeping energy expenditure in the elderly. *EurJClinNutr.* 1990;44:741–747.

10. Foster GD, Wadden TA, Mullen JL, et al. Resting energy expenditure, body composition, and excess weight in the obese. *Metab.* 1988;37(5):467–472.

11. Owen OE, Holup JL, D'Alessio DA, et al. A reappraisal of the caloric requirements of men. *AmJClinNutr.* 1987;46:875–85.

12. Pavlou KN, Hoefer MA, Blackburn GL. Resting energy expenditure in moderate obesity: Predicting velocity of weight loss. *AnnSurg.* 1986;203(2):136–141.

13. Taaffe DR, Thompson J, Butterfield G, Marcus R. Accuracy of equations to predict basal metabolic rate in older women. *JAmDietAssoc.* 1995;95:1387–1392.

14. Frankenfield DC, Muth ER, Rowe WA. The Harris-Benedict studies of human basal metabolism: History and limitations. *JAmDietAssoc.* 1998;98:439–445.

15. Feurer ID, Crosby LO, Buzby GP, Rosato EF, Mullen JL. Resting energy expenditure in morbid obesity. *AnnSurg.* 1983;197(1):17–21.

16. Osterkamp LK. Current Perspective on Assessment of Human Body Proportions of Relevance to Amputees. *J Am Diet Assoc.* 1995;95(2):215–218.

17. *NKF-DOQI Clinical Practice Guidelines for Peritoneal Dialysis Adequacy.* New York, NY: National Kidney Foundation; 1997.

Bibliography

Himes JH. New equation to estimate body mass index in amputees. *JAmDietAssoc.* 1995;95(6):646.

Tzamaloukas AH, Patron A, Malhotra D. Body mass index in amputees. *JParenterEnteralNutr.* 1994;18(4):355–358.

Appendix C
Glucose Absorption in Peritoneal Dialysis

Calorie requirements and nutrient intake calculations for patients receiving peritoneal dialysis treatment should take into account carbohydrate absorption from the dialysate.

The D/D_0 formula has recently been advocated as a more accurate method than the traditionally used Grodstein formula.[1] The D/D_0 formula is individualized for the patient's modality and transport characteristics and is easy to calculate from readily available information.[1] An explanation of the derivation of this formula is available,[1] and a comparison with other frequently used formulas has been published.[2]

Formula 1: Grams of glucose absorbed:

$$\text{Glucose (g)} = (1 - D/D_0) \times G_i$$

Where:

D_0 = Initial dextrose in the dialysate at zero hours (g)

D = Remaining dextrose in the dialysate after an appropriate dwell time (g)

D/D_0 = Fraction of glucose remaining in the dialysate

G_i = Initial grams glucose instilled:

    13 g/L for 1.5% dextrose

    22 g/L for 2.5% dextrose

    38 g/L for 4.25% dextrose

In CAPD patients, D/D_0 is determined after a 4-hour dwell from the peritoneal equilibration test (PET). Explanations of the methodology for performing the PET test are available in references 3 and 4. For automated peritoneal dialysis patients, the formula uses the cycler dwell time D/D_0.

Example: A CAPD patient uses 4 L of 2.5% and 4 L of 4.25% solution.

Initial grams glucose installed = (4 liters × 22g/liter) + (4 liters × 38g/liter)
         = 240g

D/D_0 obtained from PET = 0.58

Grams of glucose absorbed = (1 − 0.58) × 240
         = 100.8g

Calories absorbed = (100.8g) × (3.7kcal/g) = 372kcal

References

1. Bodnar DM, Busch S, Fuchs J,Piedmonte M, Schreiber M. Estimating glucose absorption in peritoneal dialysis using peritoneal equilibration tests. *AdvPeritonealDial.*1993;9:114–118.

2. Kent PS. Nutrition management of diabetes in the adult peritoneal dialysis patient. *RenalNutr-Forum*. 1996;16(4):1–3.

3. Bodner D. Peritoneal dialysis adequacy studies and peritoneal equilibration tests (PET). *Renal-NutrForum*.1994;13(4):1–4.

4. Wu GG, Oreopoulos DG. Assessing peritoneal ultrafiltration and solute transport. In: Daugirdas JT, Ing TS, eds. *Handbook of Dialysis* (2nd ed). Boston, Mass: Little, Brown; 1994.

Bibliography

Chicago Dietetic Association, South Suburban Dietetic Association, Dietitians of Canada. *Manual of Clinical Dietetics*. 6th ed. Chicago, Ill: American Dietetic Association; 2000.

Appendix D
Urea Kinetics

Urea Nitrogen Appearance

Nitrogen losses and nitrogen balance can be estimated from the **Urea Nitrogen Appearance (UNA)**. UNA is the amount of urea nitrogen that appears in body fluids and all outputs (e.g., urine, dialysate, fistula drainage) plus the change in the body stores of urea nitrogen.

Formula 1: $UNA(g/day) = UUN + DUN + Change\ in\ BUN$

Where:

UUN = Urinary urea nitrogen (measured from a 24-hour urine collection) (g/day)
DUN = Dialysate urea nitrogen (measured from the collection of dialysate outflow over 24 hr) (g/day)

and

Formula 2: $Change\ in\ BUN(g/day) = [(BUN_2 - BUN_1) \times 0.6 \times BW_1] + [(BW_2 - BW_1) \times BUN_2]$

Where:

BUN_1 = Initial blood urea nitrogen (g/liter)
BUN_2 = Final blood urea nitrogen (g/liter)
BW_1 = Initial body weight (kg)
BW_2 = Final body weight (kg)
0.6 = Estimate of the fraction of body weight that is body water. This estimate may have to be increased in patients who are edematous or lean, and decreased in the obese or very young.

- For patients who are not on dialysis, DUN equals zero. In hemodialysis patients and other intermittent dialysis patients, concentration of urea nitrogen in dialysate is low and difficult to measure, so the UNA is usually calculated during the interdialytic period. DUN then also becomes zero.
- The time interval for the collection of the parameters of UNA is typically 24 hours. However, any time interval (e.g., the entire interdialytic period) can be used as long as the same time interval is used for all the parameters (UUN, DUN, and initial and final BUNs and BWs). If desired, UNA can then be adjusted to a 24-hour period and reported as g/day instead of, for example, g/48 hrs.

Total Nitrogen Appearance

Total nitrogen appearance (TNA) can be estimated from UNA and can be used to determine nitrogen output. In a steady metabolic state, nitrogen intake will correlate closely with nitrogen output and thus TNA. For patients who are in positive or negative nitrogen balance (e.g., pregnancy or severe infection), TNA may not reflect intake. Acidosis in patients with sufficient renal function to excrete large quantities of ammonia will also alter the relationship between TNA and intake.

Formula 3: $TNA(g/day) = UNA + NUN$

Where

NUN = non-urea nitrogen (g/day)

NUN is often estimated as 4 g/day, or can also be estimated from the following equation:

Formula 4: $NUN(gN/kg/day) = 1.91 + [(0.031) \times BW(kg)]$

- In peritoneal patients, amino acids and protein are lost through the dialysate, and NUN must take these nitrogen losses into account. The dialysis amino acid losses average 0.05–0.08 g N/exchange. Dialysis protein losses are estimated at 0.1 ± 0.08 g/hr of treatment. These amounts must be added to the NUN in determining TNA.
- In continuous renal replacement therapies (CRRT), additional nitrogen losses also exist. See Monson and Mehta, Nutrition in Acute Renal Failure: A Reappraisal for the 1990s, published in the *Journal of Renal Nutrition* (1994; 4(2): 58–77) for a more complete explanation of the calculations involved in these types of therapies.
- Heavy proteinuria also increases NUN. If proteinuria exceeds 5 g/day, the extra nitrogen losses must be added to NUN.

If both nitrogen intake (calculated from protein intake) and UNA are known, **nitrogen balance** can be estimated from the difference between nitrogen intake and nitrogen output (TNA) estimated from the UNA. This will allow determination of whether a high UNA reflects a large protein intake or increased net protein breakdown. It can also be ascertained whether a low UNA reflects protein anabolism or a low protein intake. The formula, if slightly rearranged, can also be used to estimate the amount of protein necessary to maintain a steady metabolic state (i.e., Nitrogen balance = 0).

Formula 5: $Total\ N\ intake(g) = \dfrac{protein\ intake(g)}{6.25}$

Formula 6: Nitrogen balance = Total N intake − Nitrogen output (or TNA)

Urea Kinetic Modeling

Urea kinetic modeling, initially developed for the determination of adequacy of hemodialysis therapy, monitors generation and clearance of urea and allows calculation of the urea generation rate. The urea generation rate can be used to assess protein metabolism in the patient with compromised renal function or receiving hemodialysis treatment. **Protein catabolic rate (PCR)** is determined from the urea generation rate, allowing the clinician to assess the amount of protein needed to obtain nitrogen balance and reflecting protein intake in the patient who is metabolically stable. Many computer programs that determine dialysis adequacy (or Kt/V) also determine PCR.

Urea Generation Rate

Urea generation rate (GUN) is calculated using the following equations. Four separate versions of the equation are presented, each specific to a particular clinical situation:

1. Nutritionally stable, nondialyzed patient:
   a. Calculate KrUN

   Formula 7: $KrUN = \dfrac{UUN}{BUN} \times \dfrac{U_v}{t}$

   b. Calculate GUN

   Formula 8: $GUN = BUN \times KrUN$

2. Catabolic, nondialyzed patient:
   a. Calculate KrUN

Formula 9: $KrUN = \dfrac{UUN}{BUN} \times \dfrac{U_v}{t}$

b. Calculate GUN

Formula 10: $GUN = \dfrac{(BUN_2 - BUN_1)(V_u)}{\theta} + (\overline{BUN} \times KrUN)$

3. Hemodialyzed, anuric patient:
   a. Calculate GUN

Formula 11: $GUN = \dfrac{(V_{u2} \times BUN_2) - (V_{u1} \times BUN_1)}{\theta}$

4. Hemodialyzed patient with urine urea losses:
   a. Calculate KrUN

Formula 12: $KrUN = \dfrac{UUN}{BUN} \times \dfrac{U_v}{t}$

b. Calculate GUN

Formula 13: $GUN = \dfrac{(BUN_2 \times V_{u2}) - (BUN_1 \times V_{u1})}{\theta} + (\overline{BUN} \times KrUN)$

Where:
   $KrUN$ = Residual urea clearance by the kidney (mL/min)
   UUN = Urine urea nitrogen (mg/mL)
   BUN = Blood urea nitrogen (mg/mL)
   GUN = Urea nitrogen generation (mg/min)
   U_v = Volume of urine collection (mL)
   t = Time interval of urine collection (min)
   V_u = Total body water volume (mL) (See Formulas 16–18.)
   θ = Time interval between blood samples (min)
   BUN_1 = Postdialysis BUN (mg/mL) or 1st BUN measured
   BUN_2 = Predialysis BUN (mg/mL) or 2nd BUN measured
   V_{u1} = Total body water volume at dry body weight (mL) (See Formulas 16–18.)
   $V_{u2} = V_{u1} +$ interdialytic weight gain (mL)

   $\overline{BUN}$ = Average BUN (mg/mL), or $\dfrac{(BUN_1 + BUN_2)}{2}$

PCR can be determined from GUN using the following formula:

Formula 14: $PCR(g/day) = (9.35 \times GUN) + (0.294 \times V)$

Where:
   V = total body water volume (L) (See Formulas 16–18.) When no direct protein losses in urine or dialysate are present, PCR will be an estimate of dietary protein intake. In patients with substantial urinary or dialytic protein losses (> 0.1 g/kg), the direct protein losses need to be added to the PCR to yield an estimate of dietary protein intake.[1]

PCR is often adjusted or "normalized" to lean (i.e., fat-free and edema-free) body weight and is expressed as **nPCR**.

Formula 15: $nPCR$ (g/day/kg body wt) $= \dfrac{PCR}{[V/0.58]}$

Where:
   V = Total body water volume (liters) (See Formulas 16–18.)
   0.58 = Percent of lean body mass assumed to contain water

Volume Calculations

The following methods may be used to estimate **total body water volume,** or **V**. In these formulas, Weight (Wt) is measured in kilograms, Height (Ht) is measured in centimeters, and Age is measured in years. Either of these formulas can be used to determine urea distribution volume for urea kinetic modeling in **peritoneal patients.**[1,2]

Watson Method[3]

Formula 16:
For Men: $V(\text{liters}) = 2.447 + (0.3362 \times \text{Wt}) + (0.1074 \times \text{Ht}) - (0.09516 \times \text{Age})$
For Women: $V(\text{liters}) = -2.097 + (0.2466 \times \text{Wt}) + (0.1069 \times \text{Ht})$

Hume-Weyer Method[4]

Formula 17:
For Men: $V(\text{liters}) = -14.012934 + (0.296785 \times \text{Wt}) + (0.192786 \times \text{Ht})$
For Women: $V(\text{liters}) = -35.270121 + (0.183809 \times \text{Wt}) + (0.344547 \times \text{Ht})$

A formula based on bioelectric impedence (BEI) has been developed for use with **hemodialysis patients.** This formula has been shown to correlate better with total body water in hemodialysis patients as measured by BEI than the Watson and Hume-Weyer methods, and is the preferred volume method, according to NKF-DOQI guidelines, for urea distribution volume in urea kinetic modeling.[5]

Hemodialysis BEI-Derived Method[6]

Formula 18: $V(\text{liters}) = (-0.07493713 \times \text{Age}) - (1.01767992 \times \text{Male}) + (0.12703384 \times \text{Ht}) + (-0.04012056 \times \text{Wt}) + (0.57894981 \times \text{Diabetes}) - (0.00067247 \times \text{Wt}^2) - (0.03486146 \times \text{Age} \times \text{Male}) + (0.11262857 \times \text{Male} \times \text{Wt}) + (0.00104135 \times \text{Age} \times \text{Wt}) + (0.00186104 \times \text{Ht} \times \text{Wt})$

Where:
Male = 1 for males, 0 for females
Diabetes = 1 for diabetics, 0 for non-diabetics

Adjustment for Amputation

If a patient has an amputation, it must be accounted for in calculating volume. Appendix B covers the calculations necessary to correct for amputations.

References

1. *NKF-DOQI Clinical Practice Guidelines for Peritoneal Dialysis Adequacy.* New York: National Kidney Foundation; 1997.

2. Tzamaloukas AH, Murata GH, Malhotra D, Sena P, Patron A. Urea kinetic modeling in continuous peritoneal dialysis patients: Effect of body composition on the methods for estimating urea volume of distribution. *ASAIOJ.* 1993;39:M359–M362.

3. Watson PE, Watson ID, Batt RD. Total body water volumes for adult males and females estimated from simple anthropometric measurments. *AmJClinNutri.* 1980;33:27–39.

4. Hume R, Weyers E. Relationship between total body water and surface area in normal and obese subjects. *AmJClinNutr.* 1971;24:234–238.

5. *NKF-DOQI Clinical Practice Guidelines for Hemodialysis Adequacy.* New York: National Kidney Foundation; 1997.

6. Chertow GM, Lowrie EG, Lew NL, Lazarus JM. Development of a population-specific regression equation to estimate total body water in hemodialysis patients. *KidneyInt.* 1997;51:1578–1582.

Bibliography

Bargman JM. The rationale and ultimate limitations of urea kinetic modelling in the estimation of nutritional status. *PeritonealDialInt.* 1996;16(4):347–351.

Gibson RS. *Principles of Nutritional Assessment.* New York: Oxford University Press, Inc; 1990.

Gottschlich MM, Matarese LE, Shronts EP, eds. *Nutrition Support Dietetics Core Curriculum* 2nd ed. Silver Spring, Md: American Society for Parenteral and Enteral Nutrition (ASPEN); 1993.

Heimbürger O, Bergström J, Lindholm B. Maintenance of optimal nutrition in CAPD. *KidneyInt.* 1994;46(Suppl 48):S39–S46.

Kopple JD, Massry SG (eds). *Nutritional Management of Renal Disease.* Baltimore, Md: Williams & Wilkins; 1997.

Krediet RT, Koomen GCM, Struijk DG, van Olden RW, Imholz ALT, Boeschoten EW. Practical methods for assessing dialysis efficiency during peritoneal dialysis. *KidneyInt.* 1994;46(Suppl 48):S7–S13.

McCann L (ed). *Pocket Guide to Nutrition Assessment of the Renal Patient* 2nd ed. New York: National Kidney Foundation; 1998.

Matarese LE, Gottschlich MM. *Contemporary Nutrition Support Practice: A Clinical Guide.* Philadelphia, Pa: WB Saunders Co; 1998.

Monson P, Mehta RL. Nutrition in acute renal failure: A reappraisal for the 1990s. *JRenalNutr.* 1994;4(2):58–77.

Moore LW. Nutrition implications of the proposed clinical practice guidelines for peritoneal dialysis. *RenalNutrForum.* 1997;16(4):1–4.

Nutrition Support Reference Manual. Seattle, Wash: Harborview Medical Center Department of Nutrition and Foodservices; 1994.

Rodriguez D, Lewis SL. Nutritional management of patients with acute renal failure. *ANNAJ.* 1997;24(2):232–241.

Sargent JA. Control of dialysis by a single-pool urea model: The national cooperative dialysis study. *KidneyInt.* 1983;23(Suppl 13):S19–S25.

Seidner DL, Matarese LE, Steiger E. Nutritional care of the critically ill patient with renal failure. *SeminNephrol.* 1994;14(1):53–63.

Zarling EJ, Gottlieb K. Nutrition aspects of continuous ambulatory peritoneal dialysis: A review. *JAmCollNutr.* 1994;13(2):133–138.

Appendix E
Nutrition Support Algorithm

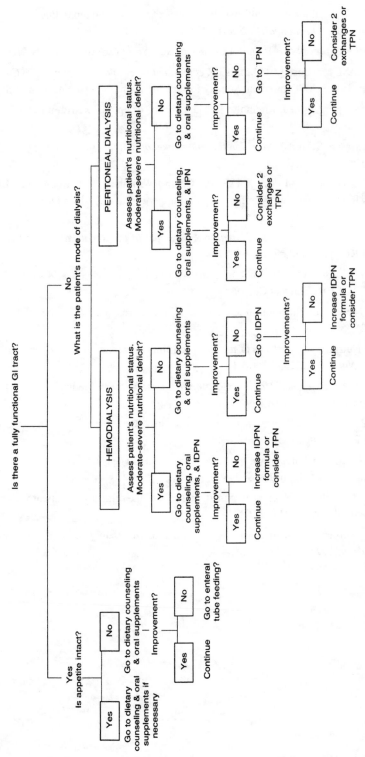

Is there a fully functional GI tract?

Yes — Is appetite intact?
- **Yes**: Go to dietary counseling & oral supplements if necessary
- **No**: Go to dietary counseling & oral supplements
  - Improvement?
    - **Yes**: Continue
    - **No**: Go to enteral tube feeding?

No — What is the patient's mode of dialysis?

HEMODIALYSIS
Assess patient's nutritional status. Moderate-severe nutritional deficit?
- **Yes**: Go to dietary counseling, oral supplements, & IDPN
  - Improvement?
    - **Yes**: Continue
    - **No**: Increase IDPN formula or consider TPN
- **No**: Go to dietary counseling & oral supplements
  - Improvement?
    - **Yes**: Continue
    - **No**: Go to IDPN
      - Improvements?
        - **Yes**: Continue
        - **No**: Increase IDPN formula or consider TPN

PERITONEAL DIALYSIS
Assess patient's nutritional status. Moderate-severe nutritional deficit?
- **Yes**: Go to dietary counseling, oral supplements, & IPN
  - Improvement?
    - **Yes**: Continue
    - **No**: Consider 2 exchanges or TPN
- **No**: Go to dietary counseling & oral supplements
  - Improvement?
    - **Yes**: Continue
    - **No**: Go to TPN
      - Improvement?
        - **Yes**: Continue
        - **No**: Consider 2 exchanges or TPN

This decision tree is intended to be used as a clinical tool by physicians and the clinical team. It is not intended to be used to determine whether a ptient qualifies under Medicare reimbursement criteria.
Reprinted by permission from Fresenius Medical Care, Anaheim, California.

Appendix F
Nutrition Support Monitoring Guidelines

Dialysis patients who receive enteral nutrition therapy (i.e., tube-feeding) or parenteral nutrition therapy, whether at an outpatient dialysis center or at home, require close monitoring of their nutritional status. The Guidelines for Enteral/Parenteral Nutrition Support of Adult Dialysis Patients delineate the level, content, and frequency of nutrition care that is recommended for patients receiving nutrition support in the outpatient setting. Laboratory monitoring is an important element in the nutrition care of this population. Following are laboratory monitoring schedules that address the chemistries that need to be monitored in patients receiving enteral or parenteral nutrition support, including intradialytic parenteral nutrition (IDPN).[1-17] It may not always be practical for the renal dietitian to solely monitor all the chemistries or for all the chemistries to be obtained at the dialysis center. The responsibility for the lab monitoring should be clarified with other health care professionals involved in the patient's care.

Table F.1: Frequency of Monitoring of Laboratory and Nutritional Data: Enteral Nutrition Therapy

Obtain Baseline	Until Stable	Stable Status
BUN, creatinine	Weekly	Monthly
Albumin		Monthly
Sodium, potassium	Weekly	Monthly
Phosphorus, calcium, magnesium	Weekly	Monthly
Serum glucose	Daily (diabetics)	Monthly (nondiabetics), Daily if routine glucose monitoring (diabetics)
Chloride, CO_2	Weekly	Monthly
Liver enzymes	Weekly	Monthly
Calories, protein intake	Weekly	Monthly
Fluid intake/output	Weekly	Monthly
Weight	Pre- and Postdialysis	Pre- and Postdialysis
Nitrogen balance, nPNA		Monthly

Table F.2: Frequency of Monitoring of Laboratory and Nutritional Data: Parenteral Nutrition Therapy

Obtain Baseline	Until Stable	Stable Status
BUN, creatinine	Daily	Weekly
Albumin/prealbumin	Weekly	Monthly
Sodium, potassium, chloride, CO_2	Daily	Weekly
Calcium, phosphorus, magnesium	3 times a week	Weekly
Serum glucose	Daily	2–3 times a week (without diabetes), Daily (diabetes)
Cholesterol, triglycerides	Weekly	Monthly
Liver enzymes	Weekly	Monthly
Serum iron, ferritin, transferrin sat	Initial	As needed
Zinc, B12, folate	Initial	As needed
Calories, protein intake	Daily	Daily
Fluid intake/output	Daily	Daily
Weight	Daily	Pre- and Postdialysis
Nitrogen balance, nPNA	Weekly	Quarterly

Periodic check of fat-soluble vitamin levels may also be indicated if multivitamin is used (e.g., vitamin A, vitamin C, zinc, protime).

Table F.3 Frequency of Monitoring of Laboratory and Nutritional Data: Intradialytic Parenteral Nutrition (IDPN) Therapy

Obtain Baseline	First Treatments (frequency as stated below)			Two Weeks	Monthly
	Predialysis	1 hour	Postdialysis		
BUN, creatinine					X
Albumin					X
Sodium					X
Potassium	X*			X	X
Phosphorus	X*			X	X
Calcium	X*				X
Serum glucose	X†	X†	X†		X
Cholesterol					X
Triglycerides	X‡				X
Liver enzymes					X
Kt/V (or URR)				X	X

*These tests should be done for the first 3 infusions of IDPN, then monitored as indicated.

† These tests should be done for the first 6 infusions of IDPN. The need for and frequency of blood glucose tests should be reassessed at that time.

‡ This test should be done prior to the first and second infusions that contain lipids.

References

1. American Dietetic Association. *Handbook of Clinical Dietetics.* 2nd ed. New Haven, Conn: Yale University Press; 1992.

2. Campbell SM, Hall J, Krupp K. *Enteral Nutrition Handbook.* Columbus, Ohio: Ross Products Division, Abbott Laboratories; 1995.

3. Chicago Dietetic Association, South Suburban Dietetic Association, Dietitians of Canada. *Manual of Clinical Dietetics* 6th ed. Chicago, Ill: American Dietetic Association; 2000.

4. Cotton AB. Enteral nutrition in the dialysis patient. *DietCurr.* 1995;22(1):1–4.

5. Gottschlich MM, Matarese LE, Shronts EP (eds). *Nutrition Support Dietetics Core Curriculum.* 2nd ed. Silver Spring, Md: American Society Parenteral Enteral Nutrition; 1993.

6. Grant A, DeHoog S. *Nutritional Assessment and Support.* 4th ed. Seattle, Wash: Anne Grant/ Susan DeHoog; 1991.

7. Kopple JD, Massry SG (eds). *Nutritional Management of Renal Disease.* Baltimore, Md: Williams & Wilkins; 1997.

8. Matarese LE, Gottschlich MM. *Contemporary Nutrition Support Practice: A Clinical Guide.* Philadelphia, Pa: WB Saunders Company; 1998.

9. *Nutritional Support Reference Manual.* Seattle, Wash: Harborview Medical Center; 1993.

10. Stover J (ed). *A Clinical Guide to Nutrition Care in End-Stage Renal Disease.* 2nd ed. Chicago, Ill: The American Dietetic Association; 1994.

11. Foulks CJ. Intradialytic Parenteral Nutrition. In: Kopple JD, Massry SG. *Nutritional Management of Renal Disease.* Baltimore, Md: Williams & Wilkins; 1997.

12. McQuiston B, Potempa L, Deguzman LG, Sackmann S. Intradialytic parenteral nutrition efficacy: A retrospective study. *JRenalNutr.* 1997;7(2):102–105.

13. Cano N, Labastie-Coeyrehourq J, Lacombe P, et al. Perdialytic parenteral nutrition with lipids and amino acids in malnourished hemodialysis patients. *AmJClinNutr.* 1990;52:726–730.

14. Cato Y. Intradialytic parenteral nutrition therapy for the malnourished hemodialysis patient. *JIntravenousNurs.* 1997;20(3):130–135.

15. Goldstein DJ, Strom JA. Intradialytic parenteral nutrition: Evolution and current concepts. *JRenalNutr.* 1991;1(1):9–22.

16. Fresenius Medical Care/NMC Homecare. *Comprehensive Renal Nutrition Support Program: IDPN/IPN Clinical Manual.* Lexington, Mass: Fresenius Medical Care/NMC Homecare; 1998.

17. Seeley L. Intradialytic Parenteral Nutrition. In: Council on Renal Nutrition of New England. *Renal Handbook of Nutrition for Dietitians.* 1993.

Appendix G
Lipids in End-Stage Renal Disease

Table G.1: Common Abnormalities of Lipoproteins in Renal Disease[1–4]

Stage of Renal Disease	Cholesterol	Triglycerides	VLDL	LDL	IDL	HDL
Nephrotic syndrome	↑	Variable	↑	↑	↑	↔ or ↓
Pre-ESRD	↔ or ↑	↑	↑	↓ or ↔	↑	↓
Hemodialysis	↔ or ↑	↑	↑	↓ or ↔	↑	↓
CAPD	↑	↑	↑	↑	↑	↔ or ↓
Transplantation	↑	↑	↑	↑	—	↔

Table G.2: Other Causes/Contributors in Dyslipidemia[5]

↑ Cholesterol	↑ Triglycerides	↓ HDL
Hypothyroidism	Obesity	Obesity
Cholestasis	Systemic lupus erythematosus	Smoking
Porphyria	Diabetes/glucose intolerance	Sedentary life-style
Dysproteinemia	Glycogen storage disease	Progestins
Progestins	Thiazides	Androgens
Corticosteroids	β-Blockers	β-Blockers
Thiazides	Estrogens	Retinoids
Cyclosporine	Corticosteroids	
Excessive intake of saturated fats	Retinoids	
	Alcohol	

Adapted from: Henkin Y, Kreisberg RA. Dyslipidemia. In: Lebovitz HE, ed.[5]

Table G.3: Intervention for Lipid Abnormalities

Lipid Abnormality	Possible Intervention
Elevated cholesterol	— Decrease saturated fat intake
	— Decrease dietary cholesterol intake (in some individuals)
Elevated LDL-cholesterol	— Reduction in weight
	— Increase soluble fiber intake
	— Exercise
	— Decrease dietary cholesterol intake (in some individuals)
	— Decrease saturated fat intake
	— Monounsaturated fats (especially in place of saturated fats)
	— Polyunsaturated fats (especially in place of saturated fats—they may, however, further reduce HDL-cholesterol levels as well)
	— Use of soy protein in place of animal protein
Decreased HDL-cholesterol	— Exercise
	— Moderate intake of alcohol (not recommended if triglyceride levels are elevated)
	— (Polyunsaturated fats may actually tend to decrease HDL-cholesterol as well as LDL-cholesterol, however, monounsaturated fats have not shown this tendency)
Increased Triglycerides	— Reduction in weight
	— Decrease alcohol intake
	— Decrease simple sugar intake
	— Increase soluble fiber intake
	— Decrease total fat intake
	— Use of ω-3 fatty acids (found in fish and fish oils); these fatty acids can also prolong bleeding time and decrease platelet aggregation, so should be used with caution. Increasing fish intake is suggested in place of fish oil supplements

References

1. Wanner C. Lipid Metabolism in Renal Disease and Renal Failure. In: Kopple JD, Massry SG (eds). *Nutritional Management of Renal Disease.* Baltimore, Md: Williams & Wilkins; 1997.

2. Attman PO, Samuelsson O, Alaupovic P. Diagnosis and classification of dyslipidemia in renal disease. *BloodPurif.* 1996;14:49–57.

3. Oda H, Keane WF. Lipid abnormalities in end stage renal disease. *NephrolDialTransplant.* 1998;13(Suppl 1):45–49.

4. Kaysen GA. Hyperlipidemia of chronic renal failure. *BloodPurif.* 1994;12:60–67.

5. Henkin Y, Kreisberg RA. Dyslipidemia. In: Lebovitz HE, ed. *Therapy for Diabetes Mellitus and Related Disorders* 2nd ed. Alexandria, Va: American Diabetes Association, Inc; 1994.

Bibliography

American Dietetic Association. *Handbook of Clinical Dietetics.* 2nd ed. New Haven, Conn: Yale University Press, 1992.

Arnadottir M, Berg AL. Treatment of hyperlipidemia in renal transplant recipients. *Transplantation.* 1997;63(3):339–345.

Attman PO, Alaupovic P. Dietary treatment of uraemia and the relation to lipoprotein metabolism. *EuroJClinNutr.* 1992;46:687–696.

Attman PO, Alaupovic P. The role of lipid metabolism in dietary treatment of chronic renal failure. In: Albertazzi A, Cappelli P, Del Rosso G, Di Paolo B, Evangelista M, Palmieri PF, eds. Nutritional and pharmacological strategies in chronic renal failure. *ContribNephrol.* 1990;81:35–41.

Chicago Dietetic Association, South Suburban Dietetic Association, Dietitians of Canada. *Manual of Clinical Dietetics* (6th ed). Chicago, Ill: American Dietetic Association; 2000.

Cressman MD, Hoogwerf BJ, Schreiber MJ, Cosentino FA. Lipid abnormalities and end-stage renal disease: Implications for atherosclerotic cardiovascular disease? *MinerElectrolyteMetab.* 1993;19:180–185.

D'Amico G, Gentile MG. Effect of dietary manipulation on the lipid abnormalities and urinary protein loss in nephrotic patients. *MinerElectrolyteMetab.* 1992;18:203–206.

D'Amico G, Gentile MG. Pharmacological and dietary treatment of lipid abnormalities in nephrotic patients. *KidneyInt.* 1991;39(Suppl 31):S65–S69.

Henkin Y, Kreisberg RA. Dyslipidemia. In: Lebovitz HE (ed). *Therapy for Diabetes Mellitus and Related Disorders* (2nd ed). Alexandria, Va: American Diabetes Association, Inc; 1994.

Illingworth DR. Treatment of hyperlipidaemia. *BrMedBull.* 1990;46(4):1025–1058.

Kaysen GA. Hyperlipidemia of the nephrotic syndrome. *KidneyInt.* 1991;39(Suppl 31):S8–S15.

Krauss RM, Deckelbaum RJ, Ernst N, et al. Dietary guidelines for healthy american adults: A statement for health professionals from the Nutrition Committee, American Heart Association. *Circulation.* 1996;94:1795–1800.

Malloy MJ, Kane JP. Aggressive medical therapy for the prevention and treatment of coronary artery disease. *DisaMonth.* 1998;44(1):1–40.

Markell MS, Armenti V, Danovitch G, Sumrani N. Hyperlipidemia and glucose intolerance in the post-renal transplant patient. *JAmSocNephrol.* 1994;4(Suppl 1):S37–S47.

Maschio G, Oldrizzi L, Rugiu C, De Biase V, Loschiavo C. Effect of dietary manipulation on the lipid abnormalities in patients with chronic renal failure. *Kidney Int.* 1991;39(Suppl 31):S70–S72.

Massy ZA, Kasiske BL. Post-transplant hyperlipidemia: Mechanisms and management. *JAmSocNephol.* 1996;7(7):971–977.

Massy ZA, Ma JZ, Louis TA, Kasiske BL. Lipid-lowering therapy in patients with renal disease. *KidneyInt.* 1995;48:188–198.

Pedro-Botet J, Senti M, Rubiés-Prat J, Pelegri A, Romero R. When to treat dyslipidaemia of patients with chronic renal failure on haemodialysis? A need to define specific guidelines. *NephrolDialTransplant.* 1996;11:308–313.

Toto RD. Treatment of dyslipidemia in chronic renal failure. *BloodPurif.* 1996;14:75–82.

Wheeler DC. Abnormalities of lipoprotein metabolism in CAPD patients. *KidneyInt.* 1996;50 (Suppl 56):S41–S46.

Zeman FJ. *Clinical Nutrition and Dietetics* (2nd ed). New York, NY:Macmillan Publishing Company; 1991.

Appendix H
National Cholesterol Education Program Recommendations for Cholesterol Management

The National Heart, Lung, and Blood Institute (NHLBI) of the National Institutes of Health (NIH) presented the National Cholesterol Education Program (NCEP) in November 1985 and released an updated version of the recommendations in September 1993.[1] The Third Report of the National Cholesterol Education Program has since been released, again updating the clinical guidelines for cholesterol testing and management.[2] These recommendations are made for the general public, however the National Kidney Foundation Task Force on Cardiovascular Disease has also recommended the use of the NCEP guidelines for patients with chronic renal disease.[3,4] For patients with renal disease, the target goals for cholesterol in these guidelines are modified slightly because of data from morbidity and mortality studies and are summarized in Table H.1.[5-8]

Table H.1: Recommended Lipid Levels in Renal Failure

Stage of Renal Failure	Recommended Levels*
Pre-ESRD	Cholesterol 120–240 mg/dL Triglycerides (fasting) < 200 mg/dL
Dialysis	Cholesterol 150–250 mg/dL
Transplantation	Cholesterol 150–200 mg/dL LDL < 160 mg/dL (0–1 risk factors),[†] 　　< 130 mg/dL (2 or more risk factors), or 　　< 100 mg/dL (CHD or CHD risk equivalents) HDL ≥ 40 mg/dL Triglycerides (fasting) < 150 mg/dL
Acute Renal Failure and Nutritional Support in Dialysis	Triglycerides < 250 mg/dL 4 hours after lipid infusion stopped, < 400 mg/dL during continuous infusion
Pregnancy (all treatment forms)	Cholesterol < 300 mg/dL

* Levels listed may be measured as non-fasting levels except where indicated.
† See NCEP guidelines for definition of risk factors.

The following is a summary of the recommendations for cholesterol management presented in the NCEP's third (2001) report.[2]

In adults aged 20 years or older, a fasting lipoprotein profile (total cholesterol, LDL cholesterol, HDL cholesterol, and triglyceride) should be obtained every 5 years. Table H.2 presents the classification of lipoprotein levels. In the NCEP's third report, LDL cholesterol is identified as the primary target of cholesterol-lowering therapy.

Table H.2: Classification of LDL, Total, and HDL Cholesterol (mg/dL)

LDL Cholesterol	
< 100	Optimal
100–129	Near optimal/above optimal
130–159	Borderline high
160–189	High
≥ 190	Very high
Total Cholesterol	
< 200	Desirable
200–239	Borderline high
≥ 240	High
HDL Cholesterol	
< 40	Low
≥ 60	High

Risk Factor Determination

Several factors (other than LDL) confer high risk of coronary disease (CHD):

- Cigarette smoking
- Hypertension (BP ≥ 140/90 mmHg or on antihypertensive medication)
- Low HDL cholesterol (< 40 mg/dl)
- Family history of premature CHD (CHD in male first degree relative < 55 years; CHD in female first degree relative < 65 years)
- Age (men ≥ 45 years; women ≥ 55 years)

HDL cholesterol ≥ 60 mg/dL counts as a "negative" risk factor, and its presence removes one risk factor from the total count.

Based on these risk factors, three categories of risk are identified which modify the goals and modalities of LDL-lowering therapy. The number of risk factors present, along with presence of coronary heart disease (CHD), determines the category of risk.

Table H.3: Three Categories of Risk That Modify LDL Cholesterol Goals

Risk Category	LDL Goal (mg/dL)
CHD and CHD risk equivalents	< 100
Multiple (2+) risk factors	< 130
0-to-1 risk factor	< 160

The highest risk category consists of the presence of CHD and CHD risk equivalents. CHD and CHD risk equivalents comprise

- Clinical CHD
- Other clinical forms of atherosclerotic disease (peripheral arterial disease, abdominal aortic aneurysm, and symptomatice carotid artery disease)
- Diabetes
- Multiple risk factors that confer a 10-year risk for CHD > 20%

Ten-year risk for CHD is determined via Framingham scoring. Risk factors used in Framingham scoring include age, total cholesterol, HDL cholesterol, blood pressure, and cigarette smoking. Framingham tables for determining 10-year risk are available in the NCEP's third report and on the NCEP web site.

LDL-Lowering Therapy in Three Risk Categories

The two major modalities of LDL-lowering therapy are therapeutic lifestyle changes (TLC) and drug therapy. Table H.4 defines LDL cholesterol goals and cutpoints for initiation of TLC and for drug consideration for persons with three categories of risk as defined above.

Table H.4: LDL Cholesterol Goals and Cutpoints for Therapeutic Lifestyle Changes (TLC) and Drug Therapy in Different Risk Categories

Risk Category	LDL Goal	LDL Level at Which to Initiate TLC	LDL Level at Which to Consider Drug Therapy
CHD or CHD Risk Equivalents (10-year risk > 20%)	< 100 mg/dL	≥ 100 mg/dL	≥ 130 mg/dL (100–129 mg/dL: drug optional)
2+ Risk Factors (10-year risk ≤ 20%)	< 130 mg/dL	≥ 130 mg/dL	10-year risk 10–20%: ≥ 130 mg/dL
			10-year risk < 10%: ≥ 160 mg/dL
0 to 1 Risk Factor	< 160 mg/dL	≥ 160 mg/dL	≥ 190 mg/dL (160–189 mg/dL: drug optional)

Therapeutic Lifestyle Changes in LDL-Lowering Therapy

The essential features of the therapeutic lifestyle changes (TLC) are

- Reduced intakes for saturated fats (< 7% of total calories) and cholesterol (< 200 mg per day) (Nutritent composition of the TLC diet is presented in Table H.5)
- Therapeutic options for enhancing LDL lowering such as plant stanols/sterols (2 g/d) and increased viscous (soluble) fiber (10–25 g/d)
- Weight reduction
- Increased physical activity

Table H.5: Nutrient Composition of the TLC Diet

Nutrient	Recommended Intake
Saturated fat*	Less than 7% of total calories
Polyunsaturated fat	Up to 10% of total calories
Monounsaturated fat	Up to 20% of total calories
Total fat	25–35% of total calories
Carbohydrate[†]	50–60% of total calories
Fiber	20–30 grams per day
Protein	Approximately 15% of total calories
Cholesterol	Less than 200 mg/day
Total calories	Balance energy intake and expenditure to maintain display body weight/prevent weight gain

* Trans fatty acids are another LDL-raising fat that should be kept at a low intake.
† Cabohydrate should be derived predominantly from foods rich in complex carbohydrates including grains, especially whole grains, fruits, and vegetables.

Metabolic Syndrome

After 3 months of TLC, emphasis shifts to management of the metabolic syndrome and associated lipid risk factors. The metabolic syndrome is closely linked to insulin resistance. The diagnosis of the metabolic syndrome is made when **three or more** of the risk factors shown in Table H.6 are present.

Table H.6: Clinical Identification of the Metabolic Syndrome

Risk Factor	Defining Level
Abdominal Obesity: Men Women	Waist circumference: > 102 cm (> 40 in) > 88 cm (> 35 in)
Triglycerides	≥ 150 mg/dl
HDL cholesterol: Men Women	< 40 mg/dl < 50 mg/dl
Blood pressure	≥ 130/≥ 85 mmHg
Fasting glucose	≥ 110 mg/dl

Management of the metabolic syndrome has a two-fold objective:

(1) Treat underlying causes (i.e., obesity and physical inactivity)
- Intensify weight management.
- Increase physical activity.

(2) Treat associated non-lipid and lipid risk factors if they persist despite these lifestyle therapies
- Treat hypertension.
- Use aspirin for CHD patients to reduce prothrombotic state.
- Treat elevated triglycerides and/or low HDL.

Table H.7: Classification of Serum Triglycerides (mg/dL)

Triglyceride Level	Classification
< 150	Normal
150–199	Borderline high
200–499	High
≥ 500	Very high

Treatment Guidelines for Elevated Triglycerides

Borderline high (150–199 mg/dL):
- Reach LDL goal.
- Intensify weight management.
- Increase physical activity.

High (200–499):
- Reach LDL goal.
- After LDL goal is reached, set secondary goal for non-HDL cholesterol (total cholesterol - HDL) at 30 mg/dl higher than LDL goal.
- Consider adding drug therapy if needed to reach non-HDL goal.

Very High (≥ 500 mg/dL):

First lower triglycerides to avoid acute pancreatitis, then:
- Very low-fat diet ($\leq$ 15% of calories from fat)
- Weight management and physical activity
- Drug therapy
- When triglycerides < 500 mg/dL, turn to LDL-lowering therapy.

Treatment Guidelines for Low HDL Cholesterol (< 40 mg/dL)

First reach LDL goal, then:
- Intensify weight management and increase physical activity.
- If triglycerides are 200–499 mg/dL, achieve non-HDL goal (total cholesterol - HDL) of 30 mg/dl above LDL goal.
- If triglycerides are < 200 mg/dL in CHD or CHD equivalent, consider drug therapy.

Further information about the National Cholesterol Education Program can be obtained from

National Cholesterol Education Program
Information Center
PO Box 30105
Bethesda, MD 20824-0105
301/251-1222
http://www.nhlbi.nih.gov/guidelines/cholesterol/index.htm

References

1. National Cholesterol Education Program. *Second Report of the Expert Panel on Detection, Evaluation, and Treatment of High Blood Cholesterol in Adults (Adult Treatment Panel II): Executive Summary.* NIH Publication 93–3096. Bethesda, MD: National Institutes of Health 1993.

2. *National Cholesterol Education Program. Executive Summary of the Third Report of the National Cholesterol Education Program (NCEP) Expert Panel on Detection, Evaluation, and Treatment of High Blood Cholesterol in Adults (Adult Treatment Panel III).* JAMA. 2001; 285(19):2486–2497.

3. Kasiske BL. Hyperlipidemia in patients with chronic renal disease. *AmJKidneyDis.* 1998;32(5, Suppl):S142–S156.

4. Meyer KB, Levey AS. Controlling the epidemic of cardiovascular disease in chronicrenal disease: Report from the National Kidney Foundation Task Force on Cardiovascular Disease. *JamSocNephrol.*1998;9:S31–S42.

5. Lowrie EG, Lew NL. Death risk in hemodialysis patients: The predictive value of commonly measured variables and an evaluation of death rate differences between facilities. *AmJKidneyDis.*1990;15(5):458–482.

6. Goldwasser P, Mittman N, Antignani A, Burrell D, Michel MA, Collier J, Avram MM. Predictors of mortality in hemodialysis patients. *JamSocNephro.*1993;3:1613–1622.

7. Avram MM, Goldwasser P, Erroa M, Fein PA. Predictors of survival in continuous ambulatory peritoneal dialysis patients: The importance of prealbumin and other nutritional and metabolic markers. *AmJKidneyDis.*1994;23(1):91–98.

8. Avram MM, Mittman N, Bonomini L, Chattopadhyay J, Fein P. Markers for survival in dialysis: A seven-year prospective study. *AmJKidneyDis.*1995;26(1):209–219.